SENIORITY

In Search Of The Best In Nursing Homes & Alternative Care In Canada

MICHELLE WEST

*Introduction by Harvey M. Nightingale, B.A., M.A., M.Ed.
President, Ontario Nursing Home Association*

Addison-Wesley Publishers Limited
Don Mills, Ontario • Reading, Massachusetts
Menlo Park, California • Wokingham, England
Amsterdam • Sydney • Singapore • Tokyo
Madrid • Bogotá • Santiago • San Juan

Canadian Cataloguing in Publication Data

West, Michelle, 1948–
  Seniority : in search of the best in nursing homes
& alternative care in Canada

Includes resource list.
ISBN 0-201-53890-3

1. Nursing homes – Canada.   2. Aged – Long term care –
Canada.   I. Title.

RA998.C3W47   1991   362.1'6'0971   C90-095917-7

Art Direction: Design UYA Inc.

Production Coordination: W M Enterprises

Typesetting: Attic Typesetting Inc., Toronto

Printing: Webcom Limited, Scarborough, Ontario

PRODUCED BY B&E PUBLICATIONS INC.

for Addison-Wesley Publishers Limited

For my father, Joseph Bucheck, who held up and held me up through the worst times of our lives. My mother and I could never have had better.

TABLE OF

CONTENTS

———

PREFACE

When John F. Kennedy was shot, I was a sophomore in high school. I was home sick that day, and my father called from the mill to tell me to turn on the TV. The night John Lennon was shot, I was working on an article. I was also working on an article when the Challenger exploded. I took a break at noon and turned on the radio to get the news, and immediately put the TV on when I heard what had happened.

And I was talking with the plumber who was up doing some work in my apartment when my father called to tell me that my mother had collapsed the night before, and that a brain tumor had been found by CAT scan.

We always remember the most important moments in our lives. For most people, the happy times are remembered most easily. But we also remember the major tragedies. And as more people in Canada get older, there are unfortunately more and more tragedies.

But there don't necessarily have to be as many in your family if you are prepared. And that is why I wrote this book.

It's a book filled with good advice from all kinds of people to help you and your loved ones make wise and informed choices about care. Only by being prepared ahead of time can you handle the emotional upheaval and the major decisions that have to be made when faced suddenly with the sort of news I was faced with.

So I hope you're reading this book *before* you need it. But even if you're already in the situation of needing care for yourself, or have a family member who needs care, there's a lot in this book for you.

I spoke with almost two hundred people before putting this book together, many of whom did not want me to use their names. But you will find the names of many caring health professionals and other people who had good advice to offer.

Should I mention the three dozen or so people who told me they would be happy to be interviewed and then changed their minds and backed out? Several people told me I should, because they are representative of how little people care about the elderly, disabled and ill among us. Oh, they all had great excuses—mostly that they didn't have time. But they should have known that when I first asked if they wanted to be interviewed.

SENIORITY

But I won't dwell on them.

I do want to thank the many people who were happy to share their knowledge and good advice generously, even if anonymously, and the people from the various groups and organizations who sent me information. I could not have done this book without them.

And I'd also like to give a very special thank-you to Wanda Elchuk, Steven Baine, Anne Smith, Wendy Cormier, Diane Freedman, Rebecca Ostry and Ruth Ellenzweig, without whom this book never could have been done.

Michelle West
Toronto

INTRODUCTION

E veryday, another family must face the dilemma of what to do with
an elderly relative who requires constant care and can no longer
live at home.

Just as we once had to face the problems of the baby boom in the
post-war period, we now have to address the realities of a fast-growing
elderly population. Currently, one out of every ten Canadian citizens is
over sixty-five. By the turn of the century that ratio will change to one
in six. These are staggering figures, and they will raise a number of
value-laden questions for social and health-care policy planners.

Governments throughout the Western industrial world all face a
growing population of elderly. One country looks to the other to see
how the individual care needs can be met on both a human and an
economical basis. As health and social-service costs continue to soar,
efficiency and effectiveness are the cornerstones of health-care planning. Today, more than at any other time in history, everyone, it seems,
is becoming acutely aware of the growing number of elderly and their
needs.

Until our own family is touched by a problem, the difficulties of
caring for the elderly may be foreign to us. The realities of everything
we have read in the newspapers begin to take on sombre overtones. All
that information we have heard on radio and television shows comes
strongly into focus. Hey, they're talking about my family! This is always
where the story begins.

Michelle West lays before us anecdotes and studies about caring for
our elderly. She surveys the bonds of human emotion and feeling in a
series of human experiences. The task of seeking out and finding the
best long-term care centre, be it a nursing home or a home for the aged, is
a voyage into something new and one for which most of us are totally
unprepared.

No one book can cover the wide spectrum of experience and
choice. But in this case, the author has developed a unique framework
for us to follow as we begin to learn what care givers can do and how life
in a nursing home can be improved.

The decision to move a family member into a nursing home is an
experience fraught with emotion, and so Michelle has provided a series

of questions and checklists to assist a family in its endeavour to ensure that the best care is found and provided.

Urging us to trust what we see and feel, she provides and promotes approaches for our questions, and by making us more knowledgeable, helps walk us through the process. Everyone is different. The family plays a vital role in helping the staff of a health-care centre understand the elderly or sick family member and his or her needs. Michelle points out that even the best of facilities cannot always meet every need or every occasion. She portrays the reality of long-term care to those who have never experienced nor witnessed it.

The author has put together, in a very balanced manner, the difficulties, the human emotion and the need for understanding, when one is looking for a long-term care facility. Her aim has been to provide the reader with information. She has succeeded admirably, by touching all aspects of the process and the experience in a truly meaningful way.

As another day passes and another family must deal with the care of a frail and elderly loved one, this book will prove to be infinitely helpful, in a way few books are. For Michelle West goes beyond the checklist approach to long-term care, and ventures realistically into the realm of human frailties, fears, and emotions.

Harvey M. Nightingale, B.A., M.A., M.Ed.
President
Ontario Nursing Home Association

CHAPTER ONE

ENSURING CHOICES AND THE BEST POSSIBLE CARE

In my research for this book, I found that the percentage of elderly in institutions is higher in Canada than in any other country in the western world. But nobody believes there will be enough beds and staff to take care of the baby boomers once they start needing care. There isn't enough money to properly fund all the care needed now, and there certainly won't be enough twenty-five or thirty years from now. With fewer and fewer children being born, there won't be enough workers to pay taxes in the future.

Many people believe that the Canada Pension Plan is almost broke, and that there won't be any money for those of us who will retire twenty-five or thirty years from now. We will be forced to rely on our own private pensions and savings. But the increasing number of people who work part-time or freelance often do not have private pensions—nor can they afford to save.

So what is the future of health care in Canada? There is no doubt that the emphasis must shift, from institutionalization to keeping people at home longer. As the health-care issue is addressed and reformed, province by province, this is exactly what is being proposed.

Most people think this is not only the answer to the money side of the question of how to take care of our elderly and sick, but also to the human side. Because most people, no matter how old, frail or ill, would much prefer to stay in their own homes until the end.

Of course this is not possible for everyone. There will always be those who are so impaired mentally that family members will be unable to take care of them, no matter how much outside help is available. And there will always be some people who are so sick that they need serious care, the sort a home setting cannot provide.

But the mind set is shifting—slowly but surely. More groups are doing more to provide the services needed to help people stay in their homes or with relatives. Friends are renting or buying houses together so that they won't be alone; one will always be there to help the other. And support groups are starting up, such as one I met with in Toronto recently.

It consists of about a dozen women, ranging in age from about sixty-five to mid-eighties. Right now, while they are vigorous, they're running around talking to people, writing letters, and doing whatever else is necessary to help bring about health-care reform. And when the day comes that any one of them is no longer able to manage on her own, she will have the other members of the group to help her. Maybe they will share houses or apartments, or maybe they will just take turns helping with cleaning and meal preparation for those who prefer to stay alone. Time will tell. But they know that they're facing the future independently, although not alone, and that is what is important. And it is this preparation that can make all the difference. Financial and social preparation for maximum independence in the later years.

I hope that groups like this are started all over the country. Because of all the things I learned while researching this book, I feel they're invaluable. They're people helping people, which is what is most needed if we are going to give our elderly and sick the care they need and deserve in the future.

I spoke with several experts in the fields of health care and seniors' rights, and want to share some of their comments.

Andrew Aitkens, director of research and communications for One Voice, the Canadian Seniors Network, which promotes the enhancement of the status and independence of older Canadians, feels: "Everyone should have full access to be as healthy, happy and productive as possible—and that means full participation in society.

"Most people who call One Voice are concerned about the federal government's policy of taxing middle- and low-income people so heavily, and so threatening the financial independence of seniors when they are on fixed incomes and have limited financial options open to protect themselves."

Steven Lewis, partner in Access Consulting Ltd., a Saskatoon-based firm specializing in health and economics research, planning, evaluation and policy development, and also executive director of the Saskatchewan Health Research Board, agrees. When asked what should be done to help care for the elderly, he said: "First, make it easy for them to remain independent or semi-independent, financially and otherwise. Second, remove the glamour from the institutional sector, and come clean about its limitations. Encourage the public to allocate its tax dollars and voluntary contributions to preventive, community-based services. People who will dig deep into their pockets for the magnetic-resonance-imaging-machine campaign, despite having no idea of whether or not it will do any good, won't give a nickel to the organization soliciting funds to enhance the demonstrably successful community rehabilitation program.

"Third, educate people to think about the choices involved in health and health care. Medicare is a wonderful thing, but its single most worrisome aspect is that, for some, it creates the impression that health is a public, not a private, responsibility—and to some extent it is, of course.

"No matter what your behaviour is, the state will pick up the tab for your bypass or chemotherapy. Now, obviously many people are sick through absolutely no fault of their own, and I don't see any alternative preferable to the universal insurance we now have for many services. But it troubles me that we will end up spending fifty or a hundred thousand dollars of public funds just to die. It's not a choice we would say is sensible, but we end up making it by default, because we are fixated with death-bed interventions and heroic technological applications, and haven't thought through the consequences. I guess what I'm saying is that I wish we learned to die more sensibly, and less expensively, so that the money saved could be devoted to services which are effective and efficient."

Lorna Reimer, occupational-therapy consultant and sessional lecturer for the faculty of Rehabilitation Medicine at the University of Alberta, says: "I don't know if the baby boomers will have a harder time adjusting to their parents' aging or needing care, but I do feel one's attitudes toward aging depend on life experiences. Society has tended to shut the aged out and minimize the extended family so that youth has very little real-life contact with the elderly. We need to change this so that the elderly again are participants in society and add balance to it.

"Baby boomers should be able to adjust by planning ahead for their parents' and their own retirement and aging. Courses and books could be instrumental in helping. It is advisable for families to discuss options for care, personal preferences, death and funeral arrangements, before the crucial decisions have to be made, so they are familiar with the alternatives and the shock is lessened."

Dr. Duncan Robertson, a specialist in geriatric medicine and vice-president of Medical Service of the Juan de Fuca Hospital in Victoria, is also the chairman of the British Columbia Medical Association's Geriatrics Committee and is currently clinical associate professor at the University of British Columbia.

"It is clear that more disabled elders are being cared for in the community than in hospital and long-term care facilities," he says. "The difference between those who are at home and those who reside in facilities is generally the availability of a care giver or care givers. So when a person has either physical or mental disability that results in her being dependent upon another person, then whether or not she has a care giver available to perform those tasks is the main determining factor in whether she can remain at home or not.

"That explains to some extent the difference between the number of males and females in facilities. Populations in long-term care facilities are female primarily because they have outlived their husbands and have no available care givers. Men of the same age are more likely to be married, and therefore they have a potential care giver at home. While much care is provided by the informal care givers, namely family members, a great deal is provided by the formal care-giving system—homemakers, home-care nurses and various other home-care services.

"When a person is disabled either physically or mentally, she requires assistance in the activities of daily living, such as shopping, cooking or personal care, in order to remain at home. The balance between individual needs and the availability of informal and formal care givers, determines whether a person can remain at home.

"People who are alone may need someone to help them arrange services. If they do not have a relative who is providing care for them, then very often it falls upon a friend, a minister or a community social worker to access the system on their behalf."

Dr. Yoel Isenberg, program director of the continuing care program at the Baycrest Centre for Geriatric Care in Toronto, says: "The price of providing round-the-clock nursing in a home setting is astronomical, and the toll on the patient and the toll on the family can be very high. It's often thought that families do not take care of their elderly relatives, but in fact proper statistics show that the overwhelming majority of families are extremely dedicated to doing this, often at a great price to themselves.

"The children of impaired individuals are themselves getting older. It's not uncommon to find children in their sixties or even seventies worried about their eighty- and ninety-year-old parents. These people are often not in the best situation and are looking forward to their retirement free of responsibility from their own children.

"I would say that the growing waiting lists for various institutional types of care represent a real crisis in the making. As I understand, they're not building any more beds because they want more people to take over with home care. But I think it's very unrealistic to assume that everybody can take over home care."

In most families both people have to work. Unlike thirty years ago when the mother was home anyway, most of today's families are just making ends meet and can't afford to hire someone to take care of grandma. There are fewer children, and a lot of them are estranged from their families. Most children, although dedicated to their elderly parents, may be hundreds or thousands of miles away and not able to pick up and move close by when care is needed.

The problems of seniors are generally chronic conditions that cause functional impairment that lasts for months or years or indefinitely. For example, a person with severe arthritis who has trouble walking may be left with that limitation for decades. These people require a variety of supports on a very concrete level every day. That may mean modification to such simple items, ones we take for granted, as can openers and cutlery; it may mean better access to buildings and subways for people in wheel chairs or using four-legged walkers and other assistive devices. And then there are the individuals with memory impairment or other kinds of mental disability.

Another problem facing seniors and anybody caring for them, whether family, friends or professionals, is the need to make plans for the future. People tend to be aware of increasing limitations and what the future brings, but concrete plans are important. This runs the gamut from planning finances carefully to making the preferences clear about the types of health care that may be required in the future.

Seniors and care givers must also plan for decisions that may need to be made at a time when the seniors may no longer be able to make those decisions.

"Every one of us should think about the fact that we're probably going to live to be fairly old and that we have to plan not only for our active retirement life, but also for our dependency years, if there are any," states Dr. Blossom Wigdor, chairperson of the National Advisory Council on Aging, member of the Centre for Studies of Aging, and professor of Psychology and Behavioural Sciences at the University of Toronto. "We may be lucky and not have any dependency years, but there's always the possibility, so we should be thinking about it. As we go through our middle years we should think about our network, our family relationships, and planning for our retirement, financially and in terms of health. Then we should think about the fact that we need to fine-tune our health-care system so that it meets the needs of people rather than the needs of government."

Asking the right questions

What about people who don't want to discuss those "what if" questions, such as "What if I need care some day?" Do they generally just say, "I'll think about it later," or "It's not going to happen to me."?

Dr. Isenberg doesn't feel that is the case. "I would say that older people tend to be much more heterogeneous than younger people, since they've had seventy or eighty odd years of unique experiences that tend to differentiate them from people with other experiences, and they've had more time to accumulate unique experiences than a twenty-year-old. There are many individuals who are all too ready to talk about these things. After all, after eighty years they've had many rehearsals of going to funerals, first of older people and then of peers, and then of people younger than they are, so they know that they've already beaten the statistical laws.

"Also, by the time they are in advanced years, people have likely had a lot of experience with acquaintances who have had a variety of illnesses and have had to have a variety of [surgical] procedures. They may have strong opinions about whether or not they would want to be resuscitated, whether or not they would want to have feeding tubes and a variety of other treatments. Individuals who have encountered this tend to develop strong opinions, but they're often not welcomed by the family. It's understandable that younger people may not want to discuss with their parents whether or not they should have a tube placed down their nose into their stomach. It may be stressful for the child, or the parent may imagine it is stressful for the child, and so it may not be a fit subject for family discussion. But if approached by a professional, that elderly individual may be all too ready to state his preferences quite clearly. I think it's important for people to clarify what their preferences are. That might reduce the stress their relatives are under when the patients themselves are no longer able to express an opinion."

Evelyn Wexler, registered nurse with a Masters of Science degree in Nursing and director of nursing at the Baycrest Centre for Geriatric Care, Jewish Home for the Aged in Toronto, has written about thinking in terms of enabling seniors to do what they can even when faced with the most serious conditions:

"The real challenge in working with the elderly is that people more readily see the infirmities and don't tap into the strengths. And even in the most severe situations there may still be some ability, and that needs to be drawn upon. I work to try to enlighten care givers to take a holistic, or integrated, approach to care. Not looking at someone as per what her disease is, and how to take care of the disease. You take care of the whole person as her needs require, and that can change and vary over time.

"The realization that you cannot completely be the master of your own fate anymore is something that we talk a lot about. But until you yourself are grappling with it, it's very difficult to fully perceive. It's the thing we probably fear the most. No matter how much education any of us has experienced, we haven't been old yet. And if you haven't been old yet, you can't fully appreciate what it is to be old.

"I think we are coming more to the realization that there is no free ride in this country anymore, and there won't be anybody else paying for us. We will be paying our own way, so obviously we have to consider that when we're looking at care options. People should be paying for their own care if they can, but not having the funding yourself should not mean you are not entitled to the best there is.

"So when it comes right down to it, someone's own financial situation should not be the factor that determines what kind of care he gets. I think everybody deserves excellent care. People who have been productive and contributed to our society for many years deserve the best of care. And somebody needs to provide the care.

"The financial bottom line should never be a care facility's or a care giver's number-one priority. The number one has to be related to care. Then you look at the situation in terms of your budget, and keep striving to do the best you can do with what you've got. If there just isn't enough money to give the care you want to give, then you've got to advocate more.

"But it's a question of priorities. How much money do we want to give to home-care programs? To long-term care facilities? How much do you want for doing transplants on babies?"

Ah, yes—priorities. Everyone certainly wants to do the best of everything possible for a loved one or friend who needs care. And if we are alone, we want the best for ourselves. This means not only being able to stay in our own residence of choice for as long as possible, but to have a really nice place to go if we do have to enter a care facility.

But given financial constraints, this will not always be possible. Even with several people committed to doing everything possible to help someone stay at home, there are extra expenses. Various types of special care cost money. If one family member has to quit working to be home with an ill relative, that costs also. It appears that only if you have money will you have a lot of choices once you or a relative needs care.

I have been told by many people that the health-care system would come to its knees if there weren't thousands of family members across the country sacrificing to provide free home care for relatives.

Can this continue? Yes, it not only can, it must. Because there will probably be much less money available to a larger number of elderly and ill people twenty-five or thirty years from now.

To sum up...

- We must do whatever we can do to ensure that the elderly and sick make their own choices and stay independent as long as possible.

- To do this, friends and family members must be committed to helping out in whatever ways are required.

- If you have a lot of money, you will have unlimited choices when you become old or sick, but if you don't, you may have to settle for what is available free or at low cost.

- Free or low-cost services may be excellent, but your choices will be limited. They will come when they have time, not necessarily when you want them to come. They will do what they can, not necessarily what you want.

- Priorities must be set, which may require sacrifice to care for someone you love and setting aside some money for the future. We cannot depend on the government anymore to do everything for us.

CHAPTER TWO

LETTING YOUR LOVED ONE MAKE THE DECISIONS

Probably one of the toughest jobs you'll ever have is making a decision about care. And you must not make it alone. It's your loved one's life, and it's ultimately up to them to say what they want done with it. If you are reading this book because you want your family to be prepared for the future, then you have the precious luxury of time, which allows careful consideration. If you're in a crisis situation right now—if grandma has just broken her hip or your mother has just had a brain tumor diagnosed—then your situation is quite different, and much more difficult.

When my mother collapsed and was rushed to the hospital, my father didn't even call me. It was only the next day, after a CAT scan and other tests revealed her brain tumor, that he admitted something serious was going on and called my brother and me.

Like most families, we had never discussed things like this. My parents had planned to sell the house in a few years and move into an apartment, but that's about as far as the planning went. And I think that's the situation in most households today.

Many people think that a discussion about the future of an aging parent involves only one question: will mom or dad go into a nursing home or not? But the issue is a lot more complicated than that, because today there are many options. So many, in fact, that until someone is terribly ill physically or mentally, or very frail, most people should be able to work things out in a way that suits them just fine.

And working things out the way people want them is very important. We've been taught all our lives that being independent is valuable, and making our own choices is what life's all about. This should not change just because a person gets older or ill.

"Just because someone can't do certain things anymore," states Dian Goldstein, a director of Concerned Friends of Ontario Citizens in Care Facilities and a teacher of seniors studies at Ryerson Polytechnical Institute in Toronto, "it doesn't mean she cannot make decisions about how they're done. Sometimes people confuse these two things."

Only in the most dire of circumstances should decisions be made for someone. These include situations where someone is so mentally impaired that he or she doesn't know what's going on, or one such as my family went through. When mother collapsed with a brain tumor, she was not capable of making any decisions. And she was even worse after the surgery. Only in a situation like this will you have to "decide what to do with someone."

"The only time families should take over and make these decisions is if the relative is in a situation where he simply cannot be involved in the decision at all, usually because he's mentally impaired," feels Patricia Fleming, manager of the Senior Support Services program for the Family Service Association of Metropolitan Toronto.

In all other circumstances, it's only fair to let people have a say in what will become of them.

"I hope that families will look at possible options," says Joan Fussell, director and former president of Concerned Friends. "It's most important to involve the person himself in the search and the decision. It's his life, and he has a right to an opinion on his own future.

"In this less than ideal world, I hope that people will show the maximum consideration and respect for others' feelings and rights. They should listen to their loved one's feelings and work to get the best care they can for them."

Ms. Fleming adds: "The very first thing the family should do is ask the parent what she wants to do, and if she wants to stay in her home. If so, then the family has to look at all the community services that are available in the area where they live, and work out what is needed and what is available and what can be afforded. And if it's realistic, based on the parent's health and availability of services, then they should set it up the way the parent wants, even if there may be some problems or risks.

"If the parent is mentally competent and wants to take the risk of staying home, then it is his right. He cannot be forced to go into a facility against his will.

"When you take someone to make an application at a care facility, they always ask him if he understands what it's all about, and if he is willing to come and live there. If he says no, then that's the end of it."

What should you do if your parents absolutely refuse to have any discussion about the future? If you're really concerned about their health and what may become of them, then you may have to call in a professional to meet with the family. It's always better to have these discussions while your parents can still make their own wishes known. Don't wait until it's too late.

"A professional can help by making sure that all family members— and especially mom and dad—understand the situation, the options involved, and the consequences of each possible decision," Patricia Fleming told me. "One way of addressing the problem is to have a family conference with a knowledgeable social worker or counsellor present, and have the whole family come together at once so that they all get the same information at the same time. It's amazing how family communication can get mucked up if one member is telling another about something.

"Particularly with something like Alzheimer's disease in the early stages. One child may deny that dad has a problem, and another may exaggerate and make him sound worse than he is. A counsellor can very often help them both to reach a more realistic appraisal of what is actually going on."

Sorele Urman, director of the central intake department at the Baycrest Centre for Geriatric Care , says: "All of a sudden you may see the power, the control and the responsibility start to shift within the family. It does stir things up. Sometimes on the surface you can manage not too badly and get on pretty well with your brother from California when you only see him once or twice a year around holidays. But when you're really having to face decision-making, and family members behave in different ways and at different speeds, it does dredge up all kinds of things between siblings.

"Of course, it could be that the son from California, not being so bogged down in the day-to-day problems, can see the situation more clearly. He may even have a bit more leverage with the parent, and when he says that we've got to sit down and work this out, she may very well be more likely to listen.

"But all of this can also dredge up things between parents and children—about how you felt when you were growing up. So it may be the best thing to find some outside support during this time."

If this sounds like a good idea for your family, there are several ways you can find a counsellor who would be happy to meet with your family. Start by calling the Family Service Association or public-health department in your area. If there isn't one close to you, contact the occupational-therapy association for your region, and they will tell you who is available where you live. You'll find these numbers in the resource list in the back of this book.

Tell them exactly what you need, and they will put you in touch with the right person. If you are alone, with no family, and you're just not sure what to do, these people will also be very glad to help you. You may need assistance more than someone who has a family, simply because it sometimes takes a bit of work to find all the help you need. It may also be more difficult to make a decision about future care if you don't have a family to depend on.

If you have the luxury of time

You can approach the care situation in an entirely different manner if you plan ahead—because the best way to handle it is to be able to discuss it with the person who may need care.

But getting people to sit down to discuss "what if" questions can be difficult.

Some professionals feel that it's best to call a big family meeting, have a big dinner and then a big discussion about what may happen to each family member. Remember, it's not only the oldest family members who may be in need of care soon. Perhaps a younger member will become seriously ill, or someone may be disabled in an accident. Once the possibilities are all on the table, solutions can be tossed back and forth and evaluated. By making this meeting a big deal, you add to its importance and get people thinking about it in advance.

Other professionals feel it's best to keep these discussions as low-key as possible. Perhaps each child can bring up just one question at a time when the timing seems right—perhaps during dinner, perhaps while shopping or working side by side in the garden. Using this method, eventually everything will probably be discussed, and certainly in a nonthreatening way.

What is best for your family? Only you can know. If your mom is very excitable and pessimistic, you may cause her endless days or weeks of serious worry if you call a big formal confab. If you tell your dad that you want to discuss the possibility of his going into a nursing home "in the future," he may get all upset and feel you're trying to get rid of him immediately—and the big discussion will turn into a big argument or worse.

On the other hand, if your family is generally quite unconcerned about the future, or deathly afraid to talk about it, the low-key approach may work better. Then you can introduce the various subjects slowly and carefully over time, so there won't be any jolts.

"How you bring up this subject can depend mainly on what kind of a relationship the parent and child have," Vic Parsons, manager of the adult program of the Visiting Homemakers Association of Metropolitan Toronto, feels.

"Sometimes just an observation on the part of the child can start a good discussion. Something like; 'Oh, I noticed that you're having a bit more difficulty doing your weekly shopping. Is that right?' or, 'I've noticed when I come over that you're talking more and more about how difficult it is to get out to the store these days. I wonder if you're having difficulties in other areas too. Have you been wondering how to solve some of these problems? Have you been thinking about the future?'

"Of course this supposes that there is a good relationship between the two of them and that that kind of comment wouldn't result in a negative response from the parent. Again it depends on the relationship.

"I think that if it gets to the point where these difficulties the parent is having are very noticeable, then one can't help but comment on it, no matter what the relationship is.

"Sometimes it's necessary to seek out a third party—a minister, a priest, social worker, or whatever. But even if you bring someone else in, it doesn't mean the parent will be prepared to talk these things over with a third party. You have to use your judgement."

Harvey Nightingale, president of the Ontario Nursing Home Association, feels that the attitude family members bring into the discussion is extremely important. Talking with a clergyman or a social worker before the discussion is a good idea.

"If the whole family is there, one person should not try to handle making the decisions solo," he says. "Unfortunately, this is often what happens. The decision and the process are often left to just one family member.

"Before any decisions are made, all the family should sit down and have a whole series of discussions about things, so the weight of the burden doesn't necessarily fall on one individual. Once everyone has had a chance to have his say, and this may include the family doctor and a social worker, a real family decision can be made. In some ways this removes the heartfelt anxiety of one individual, and the whole family can generally feel that the decision was made in the best interest of the parent."

David Wright, executive director of the Visiting Homemakers Association of Metropolitan Toronto, concurs. "Yes, the primary focus of the discussion had better be the parent. But after the parent is gone, the family members will still have to live with each other. So it's important not to end up building big walls against people who are important to you and who will maybe look after you one day."

Elizabeth Creighton, senior social worker at the Princess Margaret Hospital in Toronto, states: "As long as an older person is reasonably well, the family doesn't really think about losing her. It isn't until she gets a serious disease, like cancer, that all of a sudden they have to confront it. We don't go around looking for or rehearsing bad things in life. We have no experience in that, and we don't want to deal with it. It isn't until we get hit over the head with the reality that something is happening that we start to try to deal with it."

So think about your situation. Have a chat with the family members you're closest to and see how they feel about it.

If it's mom you're starting to worry about, approach dad in private first. Ask him if he's given any thought to what he will do if or when mom gets worse. He probably has, although he may not admit it to you. Once something happens in a family, people usually do start thinking. They may not do anything, but they usually start thinking.

Whichever approach you decide to take toward getting your family to talk about "what if," the sooner you start, the better. Once something has happened and you're in a crisis situation, you'll be very upset and it will be too late for careful thought and consideration of all the options.

The best thing about discussing the possibilities ahead of time is that each family member can make her feelings and choices known. If you haven't lived at home for a long time, your parents' thoughts about life and other things may have changed—and you may not even know. Unless you actually live with someone all the time, and sometimes even if you do, it's hard to know exactly where they stand on things. Sometimes people's ideas and ideals change radically as they age.

For example, you may bring up this subject only to find your mom telling you that she has already picked out a retirement home, or may already have plans to sell her house and move in with a friend. In other words, "Thanks for asking, but I've got everything under control already."

Or you may find her getting angry with you for suggesting that she's getting older, or perhaps even begging you to promise that you'll never put her in a nursing home.

So even as well as you think you know your parents, be prepared for the possibility of a curve ball when you open the doors to this subject.

For someone already starting to need help

If you're like a lot of people, you may live far away from home and visit only once a year, perhaps at Christmas. If you do see your family only once in a while, it may come as quite a shock to see how much mom or dad has aged in what seems like such a short time.

If there is any kind of physical illness, such as arthritis, you may notice one year that your parent suddenly seems very bad. In reality it wasn't sudden, but you weren't there to see the small changes as they occurred.

Even more devastating is seeing sudden mental changes. A friend told me that one Christmas her father was just fine, but the next Christmas she was afraid to ride in the car with him when he drove—he was easily distracted and not as alert. He missed a couple of stop signs and almost had a collision.

While many of these physical and mental changes may seem horrible to you, your parent probably isn't even aware of them. People are adaptable and tend to adjust, without conscious thought, to tiny changes as they happen. So dad may complain about his sore knees, as he has for twenty years, but may not seem to be aware that he can hardly negotiate the stairs anymore.

So if it's obvious to you that your parent can't handle for much longer everything by himself the way he always has, it's definitely time for a talk. You cannot afford to put it off. Next Christmas may well be too late.

Decisions have to be made concerning the future. Unless you sit down and actually ask your parents, you'll never know exactly what they want. But if you wait too long to bring the subject up, especially in cases of mental impairment, they may be too far gone to make their wishes known.

If this is the case, you may have to take matters into your own hands and see what care options are available and decide which are best for the circumstances. And this decision is really tough.

I asked Dr. Ivan L. Silver, assistant professor of Psychiatry and Behavioural Sciences at the University of Toronto Faculty of Medicine, and staff psychiatrist at the Sunnybrook Health Science Centre, about this.

"One of the main difficulties that people tell me concerning their parents," he said, "includes the parents' lack of insight into the nature and severity of their capacity to function. There often is discrepancy between how a parent sees things and how the child does. In other words, a parent with a disability or disorder may frequently deny the severity of a problem that may, in fact, jeopardize his very life. The children can be frustrated not being able to convince the parent that there is a bigger problem.

"In these kinds of situations, I suggest that the families take a step back. I take the pressure off them by explaining that the parent may not be able to develop insight into the nature of her difficulty, and that there may be little point in trying to convince her. Other alternative strategies may need to be considered. These include negotiating with the parent for alternative ways of providing care, or in simply not negotiating at all with the parent for the provision of care, especially if she is cognitively impaired. Children are very concerned about their own capacities to take care of their parents if particularly increasing disability develops."

Dr. Duncan Robertson feels that the first step in a situation like this is a thorough medical examination and assessment. "As a physician, the first thing I would ask of a family who is looking at care options is: 'Are any of the problems of this older person something that can be fixed?'

"A lot of the problems that occur in old age may be caused by underlying physical problems that may be treatable, and when they are treated, the resulting disability—while it may not totally go away—may be minimized. By reducing the disability, we increase the care options open to that person.

"For example, take a man in his eighties. Over the past year he has undergone a decline in his health. He used to be able to go out for a walk, and he used to be able to go out and help with the shopping, but in the past year he has gradually taken to his bed. He spends most of the time there, rarely shaves, has occasional episodes of urinary incontinence, falls down sometimes and injures himself, and his wife is getting stressed by having to provide care for a person who is is so totally dependent.

"Now if you approach that on a superficial level, you might say that the wife is getting burnt out, and that since he is obviously in need of a lot of care, he should go into a facility. If you examine it more critically, by an approach called comprehensive geriatric assessment, you take an entirely different viewpoint, asking what potentially treatable problems may be causing these symptoms. He may be taking some over-the-counter medications that he has purchased himself, or some prescribed medications that are causing these problems with his mental confusion, his falling, and his urinary incontinence. He may have an unrecognized health problem like anemia, or he may have problems with his absorption of vitamin B12, and if tests indicate that this is the problem, replacement therapy may improve his health and function.

"He may also have a depression that is unrecognized. His lack of interest in life, his lack of self-care skills, and his unwillingness to get up and look after himself, may be symptoms of depression. He may state that he doesn't feel depressed, but in fact these may be symptoms of a depressive illness that will respond quite positively to drug treatment, with the result that his health and function may be restored.

"I have a patient who, after being treated for depression, was able to resume his life with his wife in his home, and in fact was able to remain there for several years, until his late eighties.

"So my suggestion would be that people faced with this kind of decline, particularly when it is of relatively recent onset, seek appropriate medical advice from their family physician. And where appropriate, he will refer you to a geriatric specialist to see if any of the underlying causes of this disability and dependency can be treated. Even if they cannot be helped, you need advice as to the appropriate mix of services and treatments that may preserve what function that person has left, and to minimize his future dependency and disability."

In a crisis

Once something serious has happened, there may be no time to deliberate your options carefully. If dad has a serious stroke, or grandma falls and breaks her hip, some decisions must be made right away—before the patient has to leave the hospital.

Does it look like dad or grandma will be able to resume life the way it was before? This should be the first question you ask.

Many people, even though slightly damaged by a stroke, can get along just fine in their own homes with just a little help with the cooking and cleaning. Others will need more help, but can still stay home if that's what they want. But some people are very damaged, and so the decisions will have to be made by the family.

It's the same when grandma breaks her hip. In some cases, she will be able to return home without any problems. But in others, she will never be able to walk again and will need a lot of care—either in her own home, yours, or in a nursing home.

So your first step should be a serious discussion with the doctor in charge. He can only give you an educated opinion as to how well your relative will recover and resume normal activities, but it will be good enough for you to start looking into options.

Some crisis situations, such as what happened to my mother, leave no options. Even though her brain tumor was removed, she never recovered. She slowly got worse, going constantly downhill until she died six months later.

She had no choice, and we had no choice. There was no way my father could have taken care of her at home, even if she had been able to come home. Although he busied himself putting extra railings on the stairs and planning a ramp for the porch to keep his mind off things, he knew he couldn't possibly care for her at home unless she got a lot better.

When the doctor called and told him that there was nothing else that could be done for her and he had to move her out of the hospital and into a nursing home, dad was totally unprepared. Up until that moment when he was forced to confront the situation, he'd never thought she wouldn't get better.

Like most people, he had never even been in a nursing home. He talked with a couple of people, but basically he was on his own. He visited as many places as he could in a couple of days, and was forced to settle for the best of the ones that had a room available.

Could he have planned things better? Yes, he could have. He told me that they had never discussed the possibility of nursing homes, even though when she first started having strange symptoms from the tumor he thought she was developing Alzheimer's. They had been married more than forty years, and he took that commitment very seriously. Whatever happened to her, he was going to take care of her himself.

It was only after he saw how devastating this illness was and that there truly was no hope of recovery that he was forced to give up this idea and look for a nursing home. Because he couldn't accept such a plan sooner, he had only two harrowing days to find a bed for her. But even if he had longer, he wouldn't have known what to look for. He'd never known anyone else in this position before, and so he had nobody to talk to about it. Unfortunately, nobody ever directed him toward the hospital social worker.

If you find yourself in a similar situation, forced to make a quick decision for someone you love, don't despair. Dr. Silver recommends that you ask yourself what you would want in the way of care if you were in this position. If your mother loves flowers, try to find her a room that looks out onto a flower bed. If her canary was her favourite thing, try to find her a nursing home that allows birds, so she can have it with her—or at least hear other people's birds singing.

Just because she may be in a coma, or paralyzed by a stroke, doesn't mean that she is totally out of it. We do not know. She may be aware of what is going on and so, out of love and respect, we should do what we can to make her life as good as possible.

Evaluating the choices

Fortunately, most people do not have to face the sort of situation my family did. Most people have at least some time to evaluate options.

Many professionals I spoke with recommend that you make up a notebook that covers all of the options that make sense to your family and your situation. Then when you need it, everything will be ready.

If your parents are healthy, you may have a lot of time to work on this notebook. After your family discussions, write in what your parents' wishes are concerning care. Yes, even down to the flower bed and the canary. You may not know how dearly your mom treasures her canary until you have this discussion. And if that is the case, you must do everything in your power to make sure her bird stays with her.

Most people, of course, want to stay in their own homes, no matter what happens to them. And every effort should be made to work this out if possible. Many services are available to help you, and how to find and arrange them is discussed in the next chapters.

Once you decide what you want and start asking around for help, you'll discover there are all kinds of people with much to offer.

I spoke with three very caring women from York Central Hospital in Richmond Hill, Ontario. Beatrix Wilson, a registered nurse, is director of discharge-planning services at the hospital, and responsible for the palliative-care function. She is also past president of the Association of Discharge Planning Coordinators of Ontario.

Judy Raitt is a registered nurse who, for the past ten years, has been discharge-planning coordinator at York Central Hospital. She is currently the president of the Association of Discharge Planning Coordinators of Ontario and past-chairperson of the Metropolitan Toronto Discharge Planners Association.

Kathy Lamb is also a registered nurse and discharge-planning coordinator, at York Central Hospital. She is currently the chairperson of Region 7, Association of Discharge Planning Coordinators of Ontario.

As discharge planners, the main job of these three women is to help people make those tough decisions about care. They have some very good advice to offer people who are struggling with this type of decision.

"The big focus today is to get away from institutionalization and be more aware of the continuity of care levels," says Beatrix Wilson. "This would mean that people can go into a home when they are still independent and follow through that one facility with the different levels of care as they require more care, so they don't have to move from one location to another."

Judy Raitt adds, "Accessing services can sometimes be a problem. Most people think of asking their physician first when they need some kind of help, but physicians sometimes don't know how to access the services either. But talking with him or her would be the very first thing to do. Physicians are the gatekeepers of the health-care system, and most realize that they need to refer people to community services such as public health, placement coordination services, home care, and the discharge-planning department in your local hospital."

"The thing about seeking help for your relative," Kathy Lamb says, "is that it's something you have to do as a family member, and nobody really does it for you. If you don't do it, nothing happens. You are alone with your problems unless you seek help."

This is why discharge planners are so important—they make things happen. Often when people need help, they are in a crisis situation. If they end up in a hospital, then either the social worker or the discharge planner will help them.

People who are alone and seeking care for themselves probably find out about services through a public-health nurse, home-care program, home-support services or homemakers, to which they have access in the community. They seem to find out about those services by word of mouth, from their friends, possibly from their doctor, and that is probably the way most people access the services. The home-care programs have social workers who can help plug seniors into the kinds of things they may need if they require long-term care, and usually referrals are made through a hospital discharge planner.

"The key seems to be to make one initial contact, and from there the process flows like a chain reaction," says Ms. Wilson. "Once people are plugged into the system, they find out about other options that are available to them.

"The most typical problem we see is the case of an elderly patient who is well oriented but physically no longer able to manage independently. But because she is well oriented, she feels that she can stay at home, thank you very much.

"To give one example, Mrs. P. lived alone in a very rundown house with terrible living conditions. Her house was packed high with boxes, books, clothing, furniture, lots of newspapers, you name it. There was barely room for her to move around. She also had a lot of cats and wanted to go home to these animals, of course, because facilities will not allow them. So she was absolutely adamant that she was going to go home, no matter what anybody said, and no matter how much we talked to her and explained the risks. But there was no swaying this lady.

"What usually has to happen in a situation like this is that people are discharged home really to prove to themselves whether they can or cannot manage. And it is incredible how they do seem to pull together their resources and manage for a period of time—until there is a tragic incident and somebody falls and fractures a hip and has to be readmitted to hospital. It's hoped she will admit at that time that she has to go into a care facility.

"Another typical case is one where the elderly person is living alone and the family members decide to take matters into their own hands. So they will come in to see us while the elderly person is in the hospital and they will say, 'We have just decided that our mother should go to a nursing home, so will you please arrange it?'

"We go and do an assessment of the patient and get her input on the process. Often we find that mother has no intention of doing what the children think she should do, and then we have to work with the children to show them how they can best support their elderly mother at home.

"We are certainly finding that our seniors and families are becoming more demanding in what they expect and want for themselves and their relatives. Of course we try to give everybody choices, but unfortunately the level of care required often dictates where they are going to go, and based on that, the options are narrowed down considerably.

"If someone is a patient in the hospital, those choices are limited again, because the reality is that the hospital beds are needed and hospital policy is that patients have to go to the first nursing-home bed that's available. If they can be cared for at home for a period of time, but know that they will have to go somewhere in the near future, they probably can have a few more choices available to them and can take a little more time to look around to see what sort of facilities there are. The heavier the level of dependency, the less choice exists as to which facility they can go to."

I asked these three discharge planners what advice they might offer to people going through all of this. Their best advice was to check out nursing homes thoroughly. The more you tour nursing homes, the more time you spend looking at the various types, the better you are able to decide which is the best one for your loved one's needs.

They also believe you should seek out people who know what they're talking about. Family members often run around talking to people who don't know much about nursing homes, and who therefore have the worst things to say about them—people such as volunteers in the hospital and the community, neighbours who have had relatives go into terrible homes, or singing groups who have visited a home once. Even clergy may have negative feelings.

So seek out people who really do know what's what—discharge

planners, social workers in hospitals, nurses, and especially health professionals who have had a relative move into a care facility.

These people can help you make a decision better than anyone else. You shouldn't try to make a decision this important all by yourself.

Regarding the trend toward less institutional care and more home care, a lot of people feel that the baby boomers just aren't going to do it. For various reasons—time and money constraints, distance, extremely independent lifestyles—they don't seem likely to take care of their parents the way older generations took care of theirs. The main problem seems to be that there just isn't enough home care available to help people stay in their own homes. There is never enough help. Home care is constantly short of homemakers; people generally don't want to work in these types of jobs.

Nobody is quite sure what the government is going to do to ensure more home care. Homemakers need a lot of upgrading and their pay increased, perhaps by as much as fifty per cent, to make people want to do this kind of work. In addition, we have to recognize that homemakers are extremely important, and that the work they do should be much more highly valued.

Kathleen Gates, professor at the Ryerson Polytechnical Institute's School of Nursing in Toronto, feels that fewer women are prepared to stay at home and care for another person, and fewer parents want their children to sacrifice their lives to care for them.

"There has been a value shift in the direction of further personal autonomy," she says. "When I first moved to Toronto I met a woman in her mid-forties who had spent twenty years of her life caring for her elderly mother in Scotland. This wasn't uncommon there. But when the mother died, she left her entire estate to her son in Australia who never visited. This woman was left penniless at age forty-five, and I think that is one example of women being exploited. I don't think anybody wants to do this sort of thing anymore.

"There is going to be a real problem because of smaller families, increased longevity, and the increase in dementia among the elderly, because the need is going to outstrip the supply of care givers very soon. But I don't think that increased institutionalization is the answer.

"Part of the answer would be increased community responsiveness to needs. I see this happening in terms of home care in Britain. Instead of trying to fit people into existing services, they are now challenging services to tailor what they have to offer to meet the needs of clients. I don't think that's being done very well here. Here, if you fit into the service, you may get suitable service. If you don't, then you may not."

When you are evaluating care options, it's important that you visit and inspect the facilities you are considering. Be sure to check for cleanliness, but that's only one of several important things. One woman told me about a family member who went to check out a nursing home for her father. She decided to go half an hour ahead of her appointment, and she just sat in the lounge area and watched.

She saw how the nurses related to the residents, how they treated them, which is something that is really important. I suggest you also make unintrusive and unannounced visits on weekends and evenings— good times to check things out, because when you go on the official guided tour, the nursing home is up and ready for it. They only show you what they want you to see.

Nursing homes have improved greatly over the past fifteen years, but you still have to go around and check them out, because it's the attitude of the nursing-home staff that's most important, not the activities and other things that are going on there.

If your relative is in the hospital, and you're not quite sure what you should do once he is discharged, then the discharge planner is the person you need to speak with. Not every hospital in Canada has a formal discharge planning program, but still, there will be someone responsible for these duties. It may be a social worker or a nurse. Just ask.

The discharge planner will assess the patient, ask him what he wants to do, check out what resources are available to him, and provide an optimal discharge plan. The most important thing that a discharge planner can do is try to get the patient back into his own home. She knows what is available in the way of community services, and also knows all about what long-term-care and chronic-care facilities are available, if things cannot be worked out at home.

Not only do discharge planners know about these services, they know how to access them. And this is frequently the hardest thing for families to do, especially in a crisis situation. When the whole family is in upheaval because grandma has just broken her hip and won't be able to go home by herself, the last thing people want to do is spend hours and hours on the phone trying to line up services and help.

That's the discharge planner's job—and she'll be happy to help with whatever special needs you have. All you have to do is ask. In many cases, you can go in and talk to her even if you don't have a relative in the hospital.

Handling the decision
Once the decision is made, the family should stick together and put up a united front to help the parent, even if some members are not happy with what has been decided. It's the family's obligation to see that the parent's wishes are carried out.

If the decision has been made to help mother stay in her own home as long as possible, she will need the support of every family member, friend and neighbour to make a go of it. And by support I don't mean just helping her do things, like cleaning and shopping. She will also need emotional support, because the road may be tough. But if this is what she wants, everyone should pitch in and do their best to see that it works out.

If the decision is made that mother will move into a care facility of some kind, then even more emotional support may be needed. This is a really hard decision, and its implementation may be even harder. You won't help the situation if you cry and carry on as she leaves and each time you visit. If it was her decision to move, you owe it to her to support that decision and to make her remaining years as happy as possible.

Guilt is the biggest problem generally found in families when a senior has to go into a care facility. Family members have real feelings of guilt for not being able to look after their loved one, but thinking they should have somehow been able to. And there is also grief that this person has changed and is going on to another stage of her life.

Sometimes the children or spouse left at home feel abandoned or even feel as if they have lost the mother, or other loved one, forever. Of course this is not the case. She has only changed her address. She's still the same mother you always knew and loved. It may take a little more effort to keep in touch now, and to visit—but she's still there for you to love.

If there are feelings of grief and guilt, family members should talk about them. It is absolutely vital to encourage everyone to vent those feelings. They might just talk among themselves, but if necessary, an individual might see a counsellor or social worker. A lot of people hesitate to seek professional help, because they feel that they should be able to handle things by themselves. But in cases like this, a professional can really help you accept the situation.

If you can't accept it, a barrier may result, blocking a good and satisfying relationship. If your visits are wrought with guilt and other heavy emotions, you'll soon stop visiting and perhaps lose contact. And that's the worst thing of all.

The family's reaction generally isn't as bad when the loved one is going into a retirement home, where there is more independence and nicer facilities. It's the nursing homes that still have the negative concept and the stigma attached to them.

Incorrect placement—people who go to nursing homes or other care facilities when they don't have to—is a problem. And most people feel it will continue to be a problem for a long time to come. Dr. Blossom Wigdor, chairperson of the National Advisory Council on Aging, believes that currently about twenty per cent of all people in care facilities do not have to be there. With proper support, they could be at home.

And most people, until they become terribly ill or very mentally impaired, can stay in their homes as long as they have some help.

This help may come from family members, friends, or from

community organizations and churches. Where the help comes from is not the most important thing. And where it doesn't come from is just as important.

If daughters are not prepared to take in their elderly parents, they shouldn't be criticized. This is not thirty years ago when most women were home anyway, and one more person to take care of might not make a lot of difference. Most women work now, and most families need the income. Few could afford to have one breadwinner (either wife or husband) quit work to stay home with an elderly parent, and could less afford to hire someone to watch the parent during the working day.

But although people who don't want to take in their parents shouldn't be criticized, they also shouldn't make the final strike against a parent who wants to stay out of a care facility. Because other people can fill in the care and service gaps.

"Those who determine policies regarding placement in care facilities should not assume that just because families are available that they are willing to, or should, provide care for older parents," feels Dr. John B. Bond, Jr., associate professor, Department of Family Studies, University of Manitoba. "Guilt should not be used to manipulate care giving."

After you've done your best
Of course, in many cases the time comes when there is no longer any choice. You've done your best to help mom or Aunt Ethel stay in her home as long as possible, but it just cannot be done anymore.

"I see some people who hang on in their own homes far too long," Dean Duncan Abraham, rector of St. James Cathedral and Dean of the Anglican Church of Toronto, told me. "If they hadn't waited so long, they could have gone into a place at a time when they had more choice about where they could go and what they could do. They could have moved in and could have been happy, and probably had a longer life too."

Bernard Bouchard, Administrator of the Bourget Nursing Home in Bourget, Ontario feels the same way. "I support the care givers and family members by redefining their roles from villain to hero. For the most part, a care giver who places a family member in a care facility is seen by all parties as a villain, a horrible person placing her loved one in an institution. The contrary is in fact true.

"The burden when you place a failing senior in a home is enormous. The act of placement is, I believe, in most cases an act of love and courage, not abandonment. It would be much simpler for the care giver if the parent ended up in a hospital and the doctor then became the villain, and the system took its natural course. But most people don't handle it that way.

"Helping families feel good about placement is essential. They usually do not get any support, and so a lot of guilt results."

Susan M. Ellis, an occupational therapist in Toronto, couldn't agree more. "You have to learn not to judge other people's decisions.   Placement causes enough guilt as it is. Some people just cannot cope with the sound of constant coughing. Others can cope with that but cannot face cleaning up after someone who is incontinent. One husband could not bathe his wife, and people could not understand why. Finally it was discovered that he and his wife had never seen each other naked in fifty years of marriage. And he could not change now."

It's important to remember that if you've done your best, that's the best you can do. Once the decision is made—if it is by free deliberated choice or if it is forced on you in an emergency—that's the decision and it must be accepted.

If you are having problems dealing with this, get some counselling. Discharge planners, social workers and other health professionals will help you come to terms with the decisions that had to be made.

To sum up . . .

- Helping your loved one make a decision about care options will probably be one of the hardest things you'll ever have to do.

- It's much better to have a family discussion about what might happen in the future while everyone can still make his wishes known.

- Once the wishes and choices are on the table, it's the obligation of family members to do everything possible to see that they are carried out.

- If you are forced into making decisions during a crisis, your choices will always be limited.

- If you need help talking about the choices or dealing with the decisions after they have been made, seek the help of a counsellor.

CHAPTER THREE

CARING FOR THE ELDERLY
AND DISABLED AT HOME

O nly about two per cent of government health-care spending goes to home care, according to Steven Lewis, of Access Consulting Ltd. "Price Waterhouse, in its 1988 review of the Ontario Home Care Program, estimated savings of $500 million in annual operating costs, and $1.8 billion in pre-empted capital costs, by virtue of the service substituting for nursing home and acute care—and this with a budget that had not exceeded $300 million per year.

"There are dozens of studies that show how home care is cheaper than institutional care for the same disabilities/diseases with identical severity levels," says Mr. Lewis. "Potential savings are hard to estimate, but consider this: hospital utilization in Canada is, by international standards, exceedingly high, and there is a lot of room for reductions. If Price Waterhouse is in the ballpark, we can estimate that every dollar spent on home care saves two to three dollars in capital and operating costs. I think Canada could cut hospital utilization by twenty-five per cent, or five billion dollars, without anyone suffering, and this might cost us two billion dollars in home care.

"We are a nation of nursing-home addicts compared to, for instance, the United Kingdom and the Scandinavian countries. We could probably cut the number of beds by a quarter, and clients would be better off staying at home—and my estimate may be conservative. This might save a couple of billion dollars and cost half of that in increased community care. So it wouldn't be all that difficult to save three to four billion dollars a year, assuming current demographics and technology. Now, home care alone cannot achieve the savings; there has to be the political will to cut funding to the institutional sectors at the same time, to set lower targets for utilization, and so on. But if we simply adopted the best practices from other jurisdictions, we'd easily reduce beds and save money.

"It is realistic to ask people to care for loved ones at home if they have assistance and respite and other forms of support," Mr. Lewis continues. "Many people don't need to be asked—they would do it if they didn't have to shoulder the burden twenty-four hours a day, 365 days a year. Even if we paid people to look after their elderly—(themselves or by hiring help)—we'd be better off than building an expensive nursing home bed and operating it. The client would be happier most of the time, the family would feel better, and the public burden would be diminished.

"Obviously we're going to continue to need long-term care facilities, but my hunch is that in a few decades, with appropriate developments in community care, budgeting and technology, only the seriously demented will be impossible to care for at home—a few others, to be sure, but not nearly as many as now. Think of it this way: it is now accepted that the mentally competent young disabled have a right to an independent existence in their own homes, granted, with assistance. Why shouldn't the elderly mentally competent have the same expectations?

"Will some people simply refuse to deal with their disabled spouses/relatives? Yes, they will, but fewer of them will if they have assistance. Or even if they do refuse, there are alternatives to nursing homes. Sheltered housing provides a largely independent environment, with assistance as needed. It allows the elderly to maintain all their remaining capacities as long as possible rather than forcing them into a regimented environment where they're not allowed to do certain things for themselves.

"It's not a service to people to do everything for them—it's encouragement of dependency, an albeit well-intentioned erosion of dignity. I don't think baby boomers are going to become suddenly altruistic care givers in an intergenerational family structure, but most people are decent and want to help their parents as long as they are not penalized by the system for agreeing to shoulder much of the responsibility. Now, we abandon precisely those people who have agreed not to pass the entire burden of care to the public system; change in policy would do wonders for morale and intentions.

"It's short-sighted of the health system to pay for people's expensive acute care and [much of the] nursing-home care, but not for the relatively low-cost preventive community-based services. It's an accepted principle that Canadians ought not to pay directly for physicians and hospital care. Why, then, should they pay for other services essential to their health? Why, in other words, do we create an incentive for people to be sicker, and institutionalized, so they won't have to dig into their own pockets for services?

"All we need to do is calculate rationally whether it is more sensible for the government to pay a little money now to save a lot of money later. Currently, people have incentives to use increasingly higher levels of services, because the sicker you are, the more likely the services are 'free' to the individual.

"We're going to have to think a lot about these options in the future, as the number of never married and childless people grows, as the whole population ages, and the ratio of elderly to young people increases. We shouldn't assume there will be the same current arrangement of services and community configurations any more than we should assume that today's health technology will be identical ten years from now."

What does this mean for the average family in Canada? It means that too much money is being spent to keep people in hospitals and care facilities, and that it's a lot cheaper to keep people in their own homes. Even if people need around-the-clock care, it's still cheaper to keep them at home than to build and operate a bed in a nursing home or hospital.

A lot of people believe we cannot afford to keep increasing the health-care budget, and that costs must be cut somewhere. This is the central point of most provincial health-care reform studies. And as you can see from the figures quoted above, a tremendous amount of money can be saved by shifting the available funds to caring for people in their homes and away from institutional care.

"Planning and preparation for the family's aging and for involvement with the health care system are incredibly important," says Dr. Clarissa Green, associate professor at the University of British Columbia School of Nursing. "Few midlife offspring, or their parents, know what they really need to about aging, about community services, about working the system, about how dynamics inevitably change as parents and children age, about how to involve the entire family in problem-solving about the issues that come up. Too often this ignorance surfaces in the face of a crisis and exacerbates it.

"I have seen a lot of families in my practice who are overwhelmed with how little they have thought about what aging is and means, about what to do about a sick or dying parent, about old issues that crop up when a parent is diagnosed with a terminal illness, about how to handle the day-to-day family and community resources necessary for keeping an aging parent independent, how to discuss finances, dying, death, and so on.

"We live in a society where people are expected to look out for their kin. No one is asking people to care for loved ones at home. It is an expectation that is built into our society. When a family member is dependent for any reason, whether a child or an elder, the first line of defence is, and always has been, the family. Almost inevitably the word 'family' translates into 'women' because historically it has been women who have provided the unpaid labour of childcare, eldercare and nursing of sick and frail family members. Only if the family is unable or unwilling have other services gotten involved.

"As the population ages, the rapidly increasing number of seniors has heightened everyone's awareness of the expense for the government if the family responds differently to its responsibility to its kin. Given the rapid influx among women of all ages in employment, the unpaid resources for care are no longer so readily available, so it makes sense that there is both familial and government nervousness about the future. And so there should be. Midlife women are no more readily available at this time in history than are their husbands or their brothers. They are employed in paid market labour just like everyone else. It will be interesting to see how the current generations of seniors and midlife offspring—and the government that represents and responds to them— deal with this crisis situation. I know the baby boomers hope there is resolution before they become the peak of the seniors boom in the year 2030."

Andrew Aitkens, of One Voice, feels there must be an interaction between the informal and formal care, between the family and the services available to them. Since there are varying family patterns, there will be varying support needs. Many seniors are isolated because of illiteracy, or because of cultural and language differences, and geography.

Not all communities provide all services, and no national standards exist. Eligibility varies among communities and provinces. And access is not universal. In some cases, if you don't meet certain rules, you cannot get services. And in most places across the country, there are not enough services to go around. You may have to wait, or accept services at an inconvenient time. Or you may have to accept a substitute, because what you really want just isn't available. But you'll be glad to hear that things are changing!

"Choices are now increasingly being offered to clients because we know people function better in their own environment, change is traumatic, and people generally want to stay at home as long as possible," says Mary Currie, project director of the Ontario Association of Visiting Homemaker Associations.

"Choice means that clients can choose the type of care they require," she continues. "Take someone who lives alone and wants to stay in his home. He needs help with personal care, light housekeeping, and getting groceries. The exact services he needs would be determined by an in-home assessment, and he will be asked to participate in planning the services. In this way he will maintain his independence and his choices, and will delay institutionalization.

"It's very difficult for the baby boomers who are being exposed to this situation, because they already have their own responsibilities of children, jobs, community work, and so on. And the loved ones can really lay a guilt trip on them. Aging parents want their children to spend more and more time with them. Because their health is deteriorating and this frightens them, this creates additional stress for the children.

"Asking people to keep a loved one at home is realistic only if there is a solid support system in place. This includes family members who feel that they can and want to keep the loved one at home. A thorough professional assessment must be done to indicate the most appropriate location for the client and the implications of that choice. Care givers must look at the pros and cons and also make alternative arrangements if things do not work as anticipated. For example, even though you are trying to keep your loved one at home, make applications to some nursing homes. Constantly monitor your decision. If the load is too taxing at times, don't feel guilty. Try respite care.

"But remember that it is not always possible to keep a loved one at home. Each situation is unique and must be treated as such. If you can and want to try, be sure you have adequate support systems—homemakers, professional nurses, and other members of the multi-disciplinary home team. But you shouldn't feel guilty if you can't handle it. You have to look at the total picture, which includes the loved one who needs care, you, your family, and your family responsibilities—career, children, and so on.

"I personally saw my wonderful mother deteriorate mentally and physically over a five-year period. I went through the trauma of seeking accommodation and care for her. On one occasion she was at my home visiting, and she became unresponsive and exhibited signs of a stroke. We took her to hospital emergency where she subsequently became very vocal—loud, confused, disoriented. At this point she was restrained and became extremely restless. After ten hours in emergency, the doctor said he wasn't sure if she'd had a stroke, and that she needed observation— but there were no beds there.

"The only bed we could find at midnight was in a psychiatric hospital. I accompanied my mother in the ambulance to her frightening bed, and it was a horrible experience for both of us. She remained there for a week until an appropriate bed was found. The sad thing is that I was made to feel that I should have taken her home to my family in her confused and irrational state."

The point is this: if someone who works in the care field and knows what is going on has this kind of trouble, what chance do you think you have?

Well, you have an excellent chance if you are prepared and informed. Never feel that it's no use to try to get help. Help is always available. If you make the decision to keep your loved one at home and start calling around, you'll be absolutely amazed how much help is out there.

As Marcia Wargon, coordinator of Community Psychiatric Services for the Elderly at Sunnybrook Health Science Centre in Toronto, told me, "Help to families and individuals starts with information. It must be made as clear as possible to the family what is happening to the relative—causes, course, prognosis—as much as is possible with our current level of knowledge. Information also needs to be provided about what supports are available in the formal system: in-home help, respite, long-term placement, and others.

"At the same time, it is important to understand what the meaning of the situation is for the individual and family. Family members also need to gain awareness of this by exploring their relationships with each other and what each is capable of doing in the situation. Counselling about these feelings and how they relate to the current reality may be necessary to enable people to deal with the situation in a constructive way."

The first step

Without even thinking about it, many people start doing things for their elderly parents as time goes by. The son will start taking mom grocery shopping when she complains that her knees hurt when she tries to get on the bus, or that she can't carry packages anymore. The daughter will start coming over to make dinner more often, and attend to a few things that need doing while she's there. The process starts almost without thought, without consideration. But suddenly the children may be taking care of their mom a lot more than they used to.

And most people are happy to do these things for their parents, to sort of repay them for all the care they've given them. But there usually comes a time when it starts to be a little too much.

Younger people today are busy with jobs, families, hobbies, community interests, ecological concerns, and so on. While they're happy to add a few other small jobs for mom or dad, if too much is needed it sometimes becomes a problem. No matter how much a child may love her parents, there is only so much free time, only so much money.

Many people simply don't know about the various services available, and seldom find out about them until something happens and mom ends up in the hospital. Then the family learns that there are all kinds of in-home help available until mom gets back on her feet. The social worker or discharge planner will generally have a talk with the family before mom is discharged, and a home-care plan is arranged. Mom may need a visiting nurse to help with dressings or injections, someone to clean, do laundry and cook, or some kind of rehabilitation therapist.

"In our dementia outpatient clinic, approximately sixty per cent of the patients are not using available support services," says Dr. Holly Tuokko, supervising psychologist at the Clinic for Alzheimer's Disease and Related Disorders at the University Hospital, University of British Columbia Site, and clinical assistant professor of psychology and adjunct professor of psychiatry, at the University of British Columbia. "There are many reasons for this, but we feel that it's probably mainly because they simply don't know services are available.

"These services certainly aren't well publicized, and people learn about them usually only after someone in the health-care delivery system tells about them. But even then, many individuals don't realize or are unable to follow up and make contact with these services. In some cases, people may have tried different services and found that they didn't suit their needs for one reason or another. For example, most day-care programs begin after normal working hours start, so people who work have no way of getting the senior to them at the necessary time. Others have commented that having a homemaker come into the home was more disruptive to their daily routine than helpful.

"And in other cases," Dr. Tuokko continues, "some people have a large extended family, religious groups and a solid community network of friends to help them, so they don't really need services. Of course, some families refuse services, insisting that it's their duty to care for their own, and although they may need assistance, refuse to relinquish any aspect of care to others."

Don't let problems like these interfere with your getting the services you need for your loved one. Just keep calling people until you get help. As Redemptorist Father James Farrell says, "Red tape is, as always, the enemy!"

Remember, all of these services can be arranged even if mom has not been in the hospital. They're available to anyone who needs them. All you need is to be informed about them.

There are dozens of addresses and phone numbers in the resource list at the back of this book. If doing things for mom has become something of a problem for you and your family, look up a few numbers.

Before you call, sit down and determine *exactly* what the situation is. Vic Parsons stresses that when you call you should be able to give them a list of the specific difficulties mom is having. You should not tell them what services mom has asked for, because she probably doesn't know what is available and what would be best for her. The more specific you can be about the difficulties she's having, the easier and faster it will be to find assistance. If you don't mind doing the grocery shopping, but just don't have time for the other important thing mom needs, such as cleaning and doing laundry once a week, then that's what you should tell them. The frequency or list of tasks to be done can always be changed later as mom needs more help.

Start by calling the closest public-health department, or call the nearest hospital and ask for a social worker or discharge planner. Dr. Blossom Wigdor advises you to always get the name of the person you speak with, and write it down in case you have to call again. That will save you a lot of time, and prevent you from having to tell your story again and again to several different people.

Tell her exactly what you need and ask if she can help. If she can't, she'll easily be able to put you on to the right person. When people get a royal runaround, it's usually because they have not been specific enough about their needs, and so nobody knows who can best help them.

The person you do make contact with will send someone out to make an assessment of the situation. In some areas and provinces, a whole team of people will be sent out. They will fully evaluate the situation. They'll talk with your mom and other family members, and they'll determine what each person is willing and able to do. They'll look at the house. They'll ascertain exactly what is needed to help mom stay home, and what she is eligible for. After the assessment is complete, they will arrange for the services needed.

If everything you want for mom is not taken care of, and if you can afford it, you can also call private services. Depending where you live, you may find that they are better able to fill your needs. For example, she may get a homemaker for three hours a day, but you may breathe easier if you know someone is with her in the evenings too. A paid companion is perfect.

There are also a lot of small services that may meet mom's needs perfectly. One great example is SAINTS—Student Assistance in North Toronto for Seniors, a nonprofit organization funded by the Ontario Ministry of Community and Social Services, Metropolitan Toronto, the City of North York, and also through private donations. Program administrator M. Christine Hurlbut told me about the service. It was begun in the 1970s by a group of teachers and parents who wanted meaningful job opportunities for students, and who saw a need in the community. The program supplies young people to do chores for seniors and disabled adults.

"I think the real value of a program like SAINTS is that it allows the elderly to have some practical help with the tasks of running a home or apartment, which can become physically difficult with advancing age," explains Ms. Hurlbut. "We are important in helping a senior maintain some independence, and thus prevent premature placement in a long-term care facility."

Anyone who needs help can call directly, or a family member can call and arrange for help for the senior or disabled person. High-school students are available after school and on weekends to do chores like shopping, cleaning, light housekeeping, painting, gardening, letter writing, snow shovelling and other odd jobs. The fee is six dollars an hour, which is paid directly to the student by the client.

If you would like information about starting a similar service in your community to help seniors and disabled people stay independent, contact SAINTS at 35 Lytton Boulevard, Toronto, Ontario M4R 1L2; phone (416) 481-6284.

SPRINT—Senior People's Resources in North Toronto—is a non-profit organization providing home-support services to help elderly and disabled persons in north Toronto maintain an independent life-style. The agency provides meals on wheels, home help, friendly visiting, telephone security checks, respite care, transportation and escort, information and referral, home assessments and practical counselling.

Executive director Jane Moore explained that they want to offer even more services, but are governed by the funding they receive. She feels that a program like SPRINT is particularly valuable because it's a locally based community service, and people feel comfortable calling because they're right in the neighbourhood.

If you would like more information about starting a similar program in your community, you can contact SPRINT at 641 Eglinton Avenue West, Toronto, Ontario M5N 1C5; phone (416) 481-6411.

A medical alarm is one of the best investments you can make if you're trying to help an elderly or ill relative stay in her own home. These are small pendants worn around the neck, on the wrist, or through a belt loop. If mom experiences any kind of distress, say, she falls and is injured, she just has to push the button. The signal is received at a central station. A trained professional will phone to see what the problem is. If mom can get to the phone and tell him, then he'll make an appropriate response, such as calling a friend or relative to go and help her, or even an ambulance or police car, depending on the problem. If she cannot answer the phone, then appropriate action is taken, based on what is known about her history.

There are several companies supplying these alarms. You can find the ones in your city by checking the yellow pages under Medical Alarms.

Tips for organizing home care

- Get a spiral-bound notebook to record all the necessary information. Keep it by the phone or in a safe place. Be sure that all care givers know where it is.

- Record phone numbers of services you have or will use, such as grocery stores and dry cleaners that deliver.

- Keep a record of the various agencies and organizations you have contacted for help, and be sure to get the name of each person you speak with. You may have to call back later, and it will be much easier to get help if you get hold of the same person. It might also be smart to note if that person was particularly helpful or particularly difficult to deal with. Maybe you won't want the same person again!

- Also include the names and numbers of all the doctors involved in any way in the care of your loved one. Note next to each name what they do or why they are involved—dentist, dermatologist, cancer specialist, or whatever.

- Keep a list of everyone who has ever offered any kind of help. Even if someone made a simple offer of driving you to work once in a while so you can save the time it takes on the bus, keep a note of this. One day this may be just exactly what you need. Never be afraid to call and ask for help. Remember, the help was offered, so you have every right to ask for it.

- Also keep a list of every medication your loved one is taking, the dose, the time schedule, and the name of the doctor who prescribed each one. Each time you go to visit a doctor, especially a new doctor, be sure you take this list along.

To sum up . . .

- Health-care costs are rising at an unbelievable rate, and more home care is a good solution to cutting costs. It takes much less money to keep people in their homes than in hospital beds, or to build and operate facilities.

- An incredible number of services are available to help people stay independent. The trick is finding them. If you need help, call a social worker or discharge planner at your nearest hospital, and they'll take care of you.

- Never be afraid to ask for help for yourself or a loved one. Start by calling some of the people listed in the back of this book, and tell them exactly what the difficulties are.

- You do not have to be acutely ill or just released from a hospital to get these services. They're available to everyone who needs them.

CHAPTER FOUR

KEEPING YOUR LOVED ONE CARED FOR AT HOME AS LONG AS POSSIBLE

O nce the decision has been made to keep your loved one either in her own home or in your home for as long as possible, you may want to draw up a simple battle plan. I spoke with several experts in this area, and they all agree that there's a lot you can do to ensure optimum results.

How long someone can stay at home depends on several factors, the most important of which are physical ability and mental condition. Some physical problems are easily managed at home. There may be pain or fatigue, but with careful planning, these can be minimized or worked around.

Keeping someone at home is more than good nutrition, medical and dental care, and a bit of exercise—although these form the cornerstone of any home-care program. It's also making the loved one feel wanted and needed. Not only allowing him to make a contribution to his own life, but actually encouraging it.

I spoke with Dr. Duncan Robertson about this. "We have seen a change in the past few years in the nature of the population requiring long-term care," he says. "Twenty years ago long-term-care facilities were primarily alternative living arrangements for people. People in facilities for long-term care were often much younger and much fitter than they are now. Now more people can be kept at home longer.

"I think it is important that we promote the sense of wellness and activity in individuals who are elderly but not necessarily disabled. We need more projects that provide information about nutrition, drugs and exercise to reasonably well elderly people. We need to try to promote in them a sense of wellness, and hopefully this will minimize their need for services. But even if it doesn't, its benefits are in enabling people to feel more in control of their lives and able to manage in the community without necessarily entering facilities."

I asked Dr. Yoel Isenberg what advice he could offer families who want to keep their loved one healthy and at home as long as possible, and he felt that there were a number of areas to be considered.

The first area that should be addressed is lifestyle. This begins with proper nutrition and attempting to stay close to ideal weight. It's now understood that a person's ideal weight changes with age, and the old life-insurance tables that were generated thirty years ago really need to be modified for the fact that different people have different "ideals" depending on their age.

The question of activity is certainly paramount. People who are active and exercise regularly are found to benefit in a variety of ways. The heart, lungs, circulation and muscles all benefit, and so does the brain. This last, of course, includes a vast number of functions, such as mood and the speed with which information is processed and reacted to.

How much exercise is normally recommended? That again depends upon the individual. Upon how much exercise she is accustomed to and how healthy she is. And all these things depend on conditions such as heart disease. So always talk with a doctor before starting an exercise program.

It's generally believed that to have substantial benefit from aerobic exercise, individuals should have three sessions, each forty-five to sixty minutes long, a week. There is evidence that even smaller amounts of exercise can improve health. Dr. Isenberg wouldn't say that he would recommend something in the realm of only ten minutes of stationary-bicycle exercise a day, but felt that if it was all someone could handle, it was better than nothing.

There's a great range of exercises. The important thing is that a person has to be motivated to do it. If he is bored or dislikes it, he's not likely to keep at it. So it's recommended that he do something that he likes. Again, it's highly individual. If people enjoy playing tennis, that's good exercise. Or if they enjoy jogging or ballroom dancing, that's good exercise, too.

Swimming is considered very beneficial for the heart, lungs and circulation, and its relatively safe particularly in the area of musculoskeletal injuries. The only drawback to swimming is that it is not weight-bearing. It's been found that weight-bearing exercises, anything from walking and running to tennis-playing and dancing, benefit the skeleton by retarding osteoporosis, a progressive condition in which there is a decrease in bone mass, resulting in fragility. So if one of the concerns is to reduce the risk of osteoporosis, swimming would not be ideal.

If people are stuck at home, they can use their stationary bicycle or ski machine, and those are good, too. They should have a routine that they consider as important as taking medications, eating three square meals a day and sleeping at night. They're more likely to stick to such a routine if it's something they enjoy, so that may depend as much on the physical environment, or the social context—for example, dancing, or doing T'ai Chi with a friend—as on the particular exercise.

Any person, young or old, should warm up for the first five or ten minutes and then cool down for the last ten minutes of an hourly session. For walking or jogging, proper footwear is important to reduce the jarring impact on the legs and spine. Also, people should make sure that the environment is safe and there are no hazards such as a slippery surface, loose rugs, or small objects on the floor.

Seniors, and everyone in the family, should also pay attention to proper nutrition. An adequate calcium intake is important in keeping osteoporosis at bay. Ideally calcium is in the food you eat, for dietary sources of calcium, like dietary sources of everything, are better than supplements. Some individuals have problems with dairy foods, which are high in calcium, even with low-cholesterol dairy products such as skim milk. If they are not able to get enough calcium from other dietary sources, such as leafy green vegetables or sardines, they may require a supplement.

Dr. Isenberg recommends the cheapest calcium supplements available. There is some controversy regarding vitamin supplements, but his feeling is that if taken in moderation they are probably beneficial and most likely not harmful. However, people should try to eat properly. Supplements are poor substitutes for proper meals.

There are a variety of reasons for that. One of them is that supplements are often not as well absorbed by the body. Another is that supplements may provide only one particular component, and we need dozens and dozens of different macro and micro nutrients, which ideally come in foods. But generally a once-a-day little vitamin can't hurt, although it may not be necessary for those who do eat three balanced meals a day. It's also important to bear in mind that for individuals on a fixed income the cost of supplements quickly adds up.

I asked Patricia Crane, a registered professional dietitian who is a consultant for nursing homes and specializes in nutrition for the elderly, how seniors should eat to keep as healthy as possible.

The elderly who are healthy, she suggests, should start with Canada's Food Guide and use that as a tool to be sure they're getting the nutrition they need. Throughout the day they should make sure that meals include two servings of milk and milk products. Examples of one serving are a cup of milk, three-quarters cup of yoghurt, or a slice of cheese. If they are not milk drinkers, they might try to consume the milk in soups, sauces, puddings, or add skim-milk powder to casseroles and meat loaves. Cheese can be also used in many dishes.

You should include three to five servings of bread and cereals—whole-grain or enriched breads, whole-grain cereals, rice and pasta. Examples of one serving are a slice of whole-wheat bread, one-half cup of cooked cereal or a cup of dried cereal, or one-half to three-quarters cup of rice, macaroni or noodles.

Two servings of meat, fish and poultry should be included. A single serving is two to three ounces of cooked lean meat, or a cup of dried peas, beans or lentils, four tablespoons of peanut butter or two eggs.

It's also important to include four to five servings of fruit and vegetables. A single serving is one-half cup canned or frozen, or a medium-sized fresh fruit or vegetable.

Seniors need the same amount of nutrients as younger people. What they don't need so much of are the calories, because the basal metabolic rate slows with aging, and retirement usually means a more relaxed and less stressful lifestyle.

Too great a consumption of fats, sugar, alcohol and sweets leads to excessive weight gain. The best advice is to stick to the basic foods. This, coupled with regular exercise, is more likely to ensure a vigorous healthy body well into old age.

With increased fibre in the diet, such as fresh fruits and vegetables and whole-grain cereals, laxatives can be avoided.

Ms. Crane doesn't feel it's necessary to eliminate such food as butter and eggs and liver from the diet unless you have a high-cholesterol level—but you still should use moderation in the consumption of these foods. In other words, don't overdo the butter and the eggs, just use some common sense. It doesn't make sense to eliminate them completely from your diet if you don't have any problems with your cholesterol level.

She also thinks that vitamin supplements are not necessary if you're eating properly, but unfortunately many people don't. Also, a lot of seniors take an inordinate amount of drugs, and drugs can sometimes interfere with proper absorption of foods. So a lot depends on the medical condition and on the health of the individual, the number of drugs he's taking, and overall diet and lifestyle. In some cases vitamins are wise. Just check with your doctor first.

There is a danger of overdoing it, and sometimes this happens when you're taking liquid supplements, as well as vitamin pills. Sometimes people feel that if a little is good, a lot must be better.

Some seniors who live alone get into ruts with their eating, and may only eat tea and toast, or always have just one kind of soup. Ms. Crane feels you should do everything in your power to try to improve the way the senior eats, but if you just can't do anything about it, certainly a vitamin and mineral supplement is a good idea.

"People don't realize what they're doing to themselves by eating like that," she says. "They can maybe get by for a little while, but eventually their health suffers and their life is shortened."

You can get a copy of The Canada Food Guide at any Public Health department, as well as other booklets put out by each province.

"Meals on Wheels certainly meets a definite need and goes a long way toward helping people stay in their own homes as long as possible and not have to go into an institution," Ms. Crane adds. "Usually the same clients who have meals coming in are getting visits from a nurse or social worker or someone else involved in home care. But I feel that the Meals on Wheels programs are very good, and they're getting better in terms of temperature and safety of food and overall menus since more of them have started hiring consulting dietitians."

Bill Gleberzon, executive director of Meals on Wheels of Ontario, sums up the essence of the program with the following: "No one ever died of a dirty house, but you can die without a meal."

He continues: "The goal of this service is to help people avoid unnecessary, premature or prolonged institutionalization by enabling them to remain in their own homes as long as they can. And the heart of the program began with the idea of neighbours voluntarily helping neighbours to maintain their independence with dignity."

Meals on Wheels began in the United Kingdom during World War II and came to Canada in the late 1950s. In 1989, 43,000 volunteers delivered more than two million meals to 66,000 customers in Ontario alone. The majority of those receiving meals were seniors, particularly the frail, but anyone who requires the service, regardless of age can get it.

Federal and provincial governments have recently become more supportive of Meals on Wheels, because the new policy is to keep people in their own homes and out of institutions as long as possible. It is less expensive to keep people in their own homes, and it is also psychologically more beneficial for people to remain in the comfort of familiar surroundings. Meals on Wheels is the keystone of the new systems being developed to provide a gamut of community-based health and social services.

"Meals on Wheels is an essential health and social community service," Mr. Gleberzon said. "It assists in maintaining the health of those who receive meals by providing them with required nourishment. As well, the volunteers who deliver the meals provide social contact—in many cases, the only social contact the recipient may have in a day—as well as monitor well-being and safety. Volunteers are trained to watch out for warning signs of deterioration and to report back to their agencies if other assistance or emergency action is required. Friendships frequently develop between volunteers and their clientele, and the volunteers often return to visit or call after the meal has been delivered."

Anyone who needs Meals on Wheels can call directly, or a family member or health or social service professional can call on his behalf. If you feel that your loved one could be helped by this wonderful service, see the resource list for the numbers of Meals on Wheels branches across Canada.

Generally a nominal fee is charged for the meal, but those who cannot afford it will usually be subsidized. Or arrangements can be made to have family or friends pay for the meal. The fee enables the meal recipient to retain a full sense of independence with dignity. Since they pay for the meal, they feel empowered to complain about it or about any aspect of the service. And Mr. Gleberzon says that they do!

Most of the food for Meals on Wheels is prepared in the kitchens of hospitals, homes for the aged or nursing homes. In some areas, such as Calgary and Edmonton, agencies operate their own commissaries. Some agencies work with food manufacturers.

Whatever the meal source, Meals on Wheels agencies purchase the meals or food ingredients from them, and pass the cost along to the recipients.

Meals are usually served hot, but some agencies are experimenting with the delivery of frozen meals. The meals generally consist of soup, a main course, and dessert. Some programs also provide salads, bread, and such beverages as juice or milk. Frequently, special favours—gifts, cards and cake—are brought during holidays and birthdays.

Meals are delivered from two to seven days a week, depending on the agency. In most areas, meals are delivered around lunchtime.

The staff or volunteers of a Meals on Wheels agency will make an assessment of a person's nutritional needs; sometimes a doctor will prescribe a special diet. Every effort is made to provide therapeutic diets, such as diabetic, low-sodium, low-fat, bland, or pureed meals. Some communities are able to cater to food preferences and even ethnic meals. But many agencies find it difficult to meet individual requests because of the limitations of their meal sources. Others have no problem.

Many Meals on Wheels agencies also try to help their customers experience greater social contact with their peers by operating what are called "Wheels to Meals" programs. In these programs, seniors are driven by volunteers to a central location where meals are served and other social programs are offered.

I asked Mr. Gleberzon what impact Meals on Wheels has on the recipient's quality of life.

"A well-balanced meal replaces the tea-and-toast syndrome, literally eating nothing but tea and toast, which characterizes the eating habits of many seniors who live alone. The meal itself promotes health and prevents illness. It reduces the lethargy poor nutrition can cause.

"At the same time, it brings a friend, who is motivated by care and caring, into a life that might otherwise revolve around the television or radio or a telephone that rarely rings. As one frail eighty-three-year-old told me—and the thousands of others who also receive Meals on Wheels could echo her words—'I don't know what I'd do without it!'"

Of course your loved one has to be able to eat the good food provided, so dental care should be a high priority. I asked Dr. Jack Lee, manager of Dental Services for the City of Toronto Department of Public Health, and Dr. Mary Kudrac, supervisor of Dental Services, about home dental care.

"It's very clear that the most important dental problem for seniors is oral hygiene," says Dr. Lee. "Good oral hygiene is important for seniors for a variety of reasons, starting with the social implications. Without good oral hygiene people feel very uncomfortable about their mouths, about how they may smell, and so they don't interact with other people.

"For those who have teeth, bad hygiene can lead to tooth decay and other dental problems, and that then can lead to poor nutrition. You can't eat well if you don't have teeth, or if your gums hurt when you eat.

"There are also mouth problems caused by dirty dentures, and these can lead to an acute infection, which can also lead to serious illness in the medically compromised."

For seniors at home, care of the mouth is not difficult. For those who have some teeth, Dr. Lee and Dr. Kudrac recommend a soft toothbrush, and also recommend that it be small, making it easier for a person to accommodate in her mouth without gagging. People who can still take care of their own teeth should be encouraged to do so, but you may have to remind them. People who live alone sometimes just don't bother, or they may simply forget.

If your relative cannot manage the job herself, you will have to take over. When you brush you should concentrate on the area where the teeth and gums meet, and use dental floss where the brush won't reach. So if she has teeth that are close together and so tight that a brush will not get them, that's where the dental floss comes in.

For severely compromised patients, particularly the bedridden, tooth paste is not necessary. A mouth wash could be used. Ask your dentist what he recommends.

The key, though, is the brushing action of the toothbrush. For those who have a hard time holding a brush—for example, a person with arthritis—there are a number of brushing aids that can be adapted to the brush. You could put a large hair roller or a round rubber ball on the end of the toothbrush handle, so there's something large to grip. You can also buy toothbrushes with heads angled for easier use. There are also a variety of holders for dental floss.

But Dr. Lee and Dr. Kudrac recommend that if your loved one is really having problems, you should contact the occupational therapist at the local hospital. Highly skilled in adapting the environment for a person to facilitate independence, an occupational therapist would be the best person to work something out for you.

Toronto dentist Dr. Robert Edwards believes it's very important for seniors to keep the teeth they have left, and to maintain the appliances, if any, they wear. If you're caring for a senior, don't allow mouths or appliances to become dirty. He feels that fluoride is a big help to people who have teeth, and recommends toothpaste with fluoride, as well as fluoride mouthwashes. If you're caring for a senior, make sure his teeth are cleaned and that any appliances are soaked and cleaned. If you can afford it, the Interplak, an electronic toothbrush, is excellent. Arthritis affects the ability of some people to brush their teeth, and a device like this can help. The main thing is to keep the mouth clean.

If your relative's appetite has changed drastically, sometimes it can be from a sore tooth or an ill-fitting denture. He may not be able to chew certain foods. If he seems to be losing weight, it may be because of a digestive problem. If the mouth is a mess, it will affect the whole body. Everything you put in your mouth is chewed. If the periodontal tissues are infected, that infection is carried into the system.

For people who wear dentures, the dentures should be cleaned daily. You can soak them in a commercial preparation, although a solution of one-quarter cup of vinegar to one cup water is probably as effective.

But whether or not you use these preparations, you need to brush the dentures mechanically, too, otherwise a film builds up and hardens. Dentures can be brushed with a denture brush or a regular toothbrush, and a mild soap is just as effective as any of the commercial preparations.

It's very important to the health of the oral tissues that dentures be left out of the mouth six to eight hours daily to prevent inflammation, which can lead to infection. Many seniors will tell you that their dentist told them twenty years ago never to take their dentures out except for brushing, but this advice is now known to be wrong.

Dr. Isenberg adds: "Also important to maintaining a senior's health at home is a focus on his or her function. With retirement and various other changes in life, it is important to try to find other areas of activity. These may include new hobbies or new clubs where people can get together. Be sure that your loved one socializes and is active physically, socially and intellectually. It's especially important to maintain social activities at a time when your loved one sees his peers either moving away, withdrawing or dying. Physical and intellectual activity are certainly key to remaining active and independent in the community."

He also feels that grief really can affect a senior's health. It has been established scientifically that the body's immune system is impaired for roughly a year following the loss of a close relative. This has been confirmed in a variety of experiments that look at the white blood cells, which fight infection, as well tumors and other potential threats to health.

That's not to suggest that bereavement should be avoided. In fact, it's dangerous for a person not to properly mourn the loss of a spouse, or a close friend. Called aborted bereavement, it can cause problems in a variety of ways down the road. See Chapter 13—Depression among people in care situations.

To sum up . . .

- Good food, exercise, and medical and dental care are important to keeping seniors active and healthy as long as possible.

- The healthier people are, the easier it is for them to manage alone, and the easier it is for others to take care of them.

- If your loved one has trouble preparing meals, consider Meals on Wheels. Many people feel that this one service has done more to help people stay in their homes than any other.

CHAPTER FIVE

GIVING THE BEST CARE WHILE CARING FOR YOURSELF

There is no doubt about it—caring for someone who is frail or ill is one of the toughest jobs around. Years ago, when families were closer in both, physical distance and emotional ties, it was just assumed that anyone who needed help would automatically be taken in by someone else. Today you cannot make that assumption. In most cases, the decision to take someone in has to be given long and hard thought.

Forty years ago most women were at home, and even though it may have been difficult to care for both the children and grandma, at least grandma had someplace to go when she couldn't care for herself alone anymore. But today most women work outside of the home, and have a second job waiting for them at home after work—taking care of the family and the house. Most women today have no free time at all.

If there's plenty of money, you can take in grandma and then hire someone to stay with and take care of her twenty-four hours a day. But most people do not have that kind of money. So if a family decides to take her in, it seems as if a third job has been added to the other two women are already doing.

And yet, an amazing number of people are doing just this. In fact, *most* of the care being given in Canada today is being given by relatives—not by care facilities. And this number will be increasing as health-care reform takes place across the country and more emphasis is put on keeping people at home rather than in institutions.

The people I spoke with while researching this book were beside themselves with praise for people who handle the difficult job of care giving—and do it well. "The work of relatives for elderly members of the family is heroic, inspiring and worthy of imitation," says Father James Farrell.

But unfortunately too many people do it *too* well—they give too much of themselves in their desire to give to others. This can lead to emotional stress, and in severe cases, can create a second patient—the care giver.

"Family members caring for an elderly relative at home must find ways to meet their own needs, as well as those of the person they are caring for," advises Marlien McKay, occupational therapist and acting rehabilitation consultant for the public-health and medical-services division of the New Brunswick Department of Health and Community Services. "Services cannot just be directed toward the ill person. The care giver must be supported in achieving a balance of work, rest and play in her life also."

Kathleen Gates says: "When I talk with women who are considering taking in their elderly mothers or fathers, I try to help them explore the different options they have, including looking at what the other siblings can do. I find that often a designated care giver doesn't explore these options very readily, but it can be helpful. I show her the consequences of the various options on the parent, because it's not just the care giver who can have problems if the relationship is poor or if someone is feeling resentful."

Elizabeth Creighton, senior social worker at Princess Margaret Hospital in Toronto, believes many older people don't want to be a burden. "They also don't want to disrupt the lives of their children. They see that their children are leading very busy lives, with children of their own, teenagers running around, jobs, spouse. There probably isn't much extra room in the house for mom to move in. Money may be tight. The children may be offering to give the best love and support in the world, but it's a chaotic setting for mom to move into, and she may find it very distressing."

Vic Parsons adds: "I think people need to understand—and to make it clear to their senior relatives—that asking for help does not necessarily make a burden. It can be a very positive problem solving mechanism. Perhaps mom may be asking to move in with you, but what she really wants is for you to help her find a way she can stay in her own home."

Dean Duncan Abraham thinks it's true that parents quite understandably don't like to impose on their children. "But," he feels, "children have to recognize that this is an excellent opportunity for them to repay their parents for all the love and concern they've showed for them throughout the early years." And they can repay them not only by taking them in, but also by helping them stay in their own homes.

Family members who want to help their elderly relatives should try to find an advocate among anyone providing services to them, since these people often know the system and can really help with accessing information and support. Find someone who is especially helpful to you, someone you can really communicate with, and then don't be afraid to ask for what you need. Remember that these people are in these jobs to help you keep your relative at home, so never hesitate to ask for assistance if you have a special problem.

Families should be active participants in defining their needs and solving problems. Don't just accept a solution because some professional recommended it. The most important members of the team are the family and the senior. What they want should come first.

Join a seniors organization or subscribe to newspapers and magazines for seniors to learn about eldercare. Consciously develop a support-system network in your community made up of relatives, neighbours, friends and professionals. Accept and ask for help!

You'll probably find that a lot of people will say something like, "Just call me if you need anything." By saying this, a person probably feels that she's made the offer and can rest with a clear conscience. But you have to learn to ask for the help you need. So when you hear a phrase like that, you should immediately say, "Oh, thank you! Yes, I need a casserole for Tuesday so I can go to my art class." Or, "Yes, thank you! I'll need someone to stay with dad for about three hours next Thursday so I can get all the shopping done."

Have expectations for and give responsibilities to your elderly relative. He should be treated like one of the family, not a guest. Let him do whatever he can—put away silverware, take out newspapers, make beds, and so on.

Ensure that your needs as care giver are balanced among the physical, social, psychological and spiritual. Take a break. Use respite care if it is available. You must ensure your own well-being in order to care for others.

If you burn out, you'll become a patient too.

As Evelyn Wexler told me, "It can be very tough caring for an elderly loved one at home. But you have to take advantage of the services and support groups that are available. If there's nothing available, could you help or encourage somebody to start one? Is there a resource in the community that could be doing that? Is there a professional social worker? Is there a mental-health nurse? Is there somebody in education or somebody who could be providing some support on a one-to-one basis, or perhaps in a group?

"There's no question. I think that money can't buy you happiness, but it can buy an awful lot of help. There is truth to that."

In some cases the family can create conditions that seem to make seniors more frail. They can cloister them and overprotect them. I've talked to people who feel that you should by all means encourage the seniors to do as much as they can possibly do, to keep as active as possible for as long as possible.

"It's important for the senior's care givers to have their own support," says Dr. Yoel Isenberg. "In fact there have been some studies that suggest that support should be directed more to care givers than to the patient himself. Think of a man with Alzheimer's disease who is somewhat oblivious to his position, but whose wife is carrying a tremendous burden. If that wife does not get adequate support, then when a crisis erupts in her life, say, a physical illness of her own, overnight one can be presented with two patients.

"The same is true for adult children who are caring for their parents and anybody else. It may be a kind neighbour, a brother or sister, friend, niece or nephew. Frequently it's a daughter-in-law. These people need to have support. They sometimes need to have relief or a break in their routine, and there are a variety of respite programs that are available for this purpose. This is very important in maintaining an individual with increasing disabilities in the community."

As Dr. Duncan Robertson told me, "Sometimes people make the mistake of trying to provide all the care themselves when there are services available that would give them some respite or relief from the burdens of care giving. I suggest to people that they learn what resources are available in their area, and with a knowledgeable health professional—a physician, home-care nurse or home-care coordinator—try to assemble a mixture of both family care and paid care services, which will enable them to continue to provide care for the elderly or disabled person at home for as long as possible.

"A wife may have difficulty attending to the personal care of her husband, yet have no difficulty providing meals, support and supervision during the day. And so, to have a home-care person come in for an hour or two a day to assist with bathing and dressing could well enable the wife continue in a care-giving role."

Dr. M. Oluwafemi Agbayewa, associate professor and head of the Department of Psychiatry, Prince George Regional Hospital, B.C. agrees. "You can only provide adequate care for someone when you have a fallback position. In other words, it is easier to provide care in the community when you know that if you can no longer do it, somebody will assist you and take the problem off your hands for a short time, or help you in some other way. This means that we have to have professionals available in the community, as well as hospital beds and respite beds available in facilities, so that when the family can no longer deal with the problem, there will be someone to help and some place for the senior to go for a while. We need to look at all the different levels of care and how they relate to each other."

I asked Dr. Robertson about the hardest thing for care givers to handle. "I feel that coping with very ambivalent feelings when you are seeking admission to a long-term care facility for a family member is probably the most difficult problem facing the spouse or the relative of the person being admitted to a nursing home or long-term-care hospital.

"Very often that care giver has been providing care or support for a patient for months or sometimes even years before admission. She has seen deterioration in the physical or mental health of her loved one, and may have reached the point where she can no longer manage to provide care at home with the resources available in the community.

"So inevitably, there is some sense of failure, for being unable to continue to provide care for her relative at home. Very often the factor that has led to the nursing home or long-term-home admission has been a significant deterioration of the person's health, and very often a change in the relationship between the care giver and the person receiving care. So all the feelings that surround the admission are perhaps the most difficult thing that people have to face."

Signs that you're burning out

If you've been caring for someone for a while, the stress may be starting to get to you. Sheila Smyth, a social worker, central intake department at the Baycrest Centre for Geriatric Care, tells you to watch for the following warning signs: feeling stuck, overwhelmed, powerless, feeling everything is "on hold," that the care giving is interfering seriously with other relationships and activities, such as work, children, marriage. For example, the daughter may feel guilty going to a movie and can't enjoy it because she knows mom is sitting at home all alone. She has to find some support somewhere.

If you see these signs, take action. Get help, get away, don't seek one all-encompassing solution, but rather, seek pieces of help. Most people can handle each individual thing by itself, but an accumulation seems overwhelming. Establish what you can and cannot do. Different people have different tolerances. You have to learn to accept yours without guilt.

The care the frail elderly need now is different from in the past. People are older and frailer, and tend to have longer, chronic debilitating illnesses. Your typical grandma is no longer sixty-two and able to help out until she dies suddenly of a heart attack. Both care givers and care recipients are older, and there can also be multiple care recipients for one care giver.

Differentiate between care and work. Many families now give a lot of care, but may delegate some of the actual work. Anyone can wash dishes and floors and do the laundry. Save your energy and strength for the really important things: communicating, loving and supporting mom.

What can be done to help care givers and their parents ensure a good life?

Marlien McKay suggests the following:

1. Ensure you balance all four areas of life—the physical, psychological, social and spiritual. Don't just give attention to physical-care needs. For example, if mother wants to go Christmas shopping, but you feel the cold will be harmful, stop and remember to think of meeting equally important psychological, social, spiritual needs.

2. Encourage care givers and seniors to stay involved in activities and with people that meet all four needs. Physical care should never be considered the only or most important need.

3. Allow risks and choice. Social and emotional well-being are as important as physical safety.

4. People receiving care have needs no different from anyone else's. What is required is that special attention be given so that these needs are not underemphasized in the desire to give physical care. All people, especially those who have physical and mental limitations, need to actively participate in meaningful activities. Participation promotes self-worth and maintains ability.

How can these needs be met?

1. Provide choice. First, allow privacy—environmental (room dividers) and scheduling (time alone to putter in the kitchen or talk on the phone); second, allow activities/roles—grandma could be the official gardener, cookie baker.

2. Have expectations for maximum independence. Caring for someone does not necessarily mean doing everything for them.

3. Allow time to encourage independence. It may take longer for the senior to get up on her own, but if she can, this should be encouraged.

4. Share the household responsibilities, such as watering the plants.

Lorna Reimer, occupational-therapist consultant, adds: "The best advice I can offer to someone who is caring for a relative at home is to contact her local home-care program or public-health unit. If these are not available, look to places that specialize in or cater to seniors, such as geriatric hospitals, homes or rehab centres, senior advisory boards, societies for seniors or the retired, gerontology programs at universities or community colleges. And don't forget about calling in an occupational therapist, as our primary focus is to assist people to function as independently as possible whatever the life situation. Occupational therapists are well qualified to provide help and assistance to anyone caring for a relative at home."

To sum up . . .

- Taking care of a loved one should not be seen as a burden. It should be considered an opportunity to repay a parent for all the love and care she has given you all of your life.

- Never try to take care of someone by yourself. Enlist the help of all other relatives, as well as friends and neighbours. Divide up the work so that no one person gets burnt out.

- If you feel under too much stress, help is available. Call a social worker, occupational therapist or discharge planner, and ask for what you need. They're there to help.

CHAPTER SIX

EMOTIONAL ASPECTS OF CARE

Unless someone is too mentally impaired to be aware of what's going on, it's devastating to wake up one morning with the realization "I just can't take care of myself anymore."

We need care when we are very young, but we don't think about why we need it. We just accept it. It's only later, after we have learned to take care of ourselves and become independent, that needing care again can be so difficult to accept.

Being cared for by others is something not all of us will have to face, but it is something all of us can certainly sympathize with.

People who are independent are truly valued in society today. "Standing on our own two feet" is highly regarded. People who cannot take care of themselves are considered weak or deficient in some way, even if it's not their fault they need help. Only small children seem to get away with it uncriticized.

The way society looks at people who cannot take care of themselves is only part of the emotional burden that must be worked through once someone starts to need care. For many people who have valued independence and freedom above all else, it may be almost impossible to accept.

For the family, seeing that mom or dad can no longer handle everything can be quite a shock, too.

Marcia Wargon believes that families usually respond to a crisis issue in the same style they have developed over time. "Pre-existing relationships colour the way in which members respond to the situation," she says. "Consequently, each family's response is unique and needs to be viewed as such. There are, of course, certain universal feelings and attributes, and the nature of the system of services has an impact on the response.

"For most families and individuals there is a tendency to assume everything will go well. Few people plan for being cognitively impaired or physically frail. As a result, spouses or children faced with such a situation often have to deal with very practical issues such as finances and help with the activities of daily living, as well as with the emotional stress of acknowledging the deterioration of the relative and their own sense of loss or anger or frustration, once it has happened.

"For the most part, people do not recognize or admit the amount of care a relative needs until it begins to affect their own lives. It is not uncommon for one spouse to 'cover' for the failing spouse, and only when the well person is removed from the scene does it become clear how incapable the other is. It obviously is difficult for a spouse or child, whose relationship to the declining person is one of dependence or great respect, to allow himself to admit what is happening and admit the need for help. Children may not feel comfortable looking into their parents' bedroom, bathroom or even kitchen, so they do not really know the extent to which mother or father is failing."

Children who live far away from their parents and perhaps only visit once or twice a year are generally quite taken aback when they see how much a parent has changed in the time between visits. But I would suspect that most do not say anything.

My father did not call me and my brother the night mother collapsed, but only the next day, after tests found her brain tumor. And then, a couple of weeks later, he told us that she had fallen a few times before, once hurting her wrist quite badly.

Although we spoke on the phone every second Sunday, I never knew anything was wrong, because they never told me anything was wrong. Were they just trying to spare me worry, because there was little I could do from so far away, or were they denying the possibility that anything was seriously wrong?

It seems to be very important to parents not to become a "burden" to their children in any way. They do not want to interfere in their children's lives, and they do not want anyone to think they are not as independent as they used to be.

Weren't many of us raised thinking our parents could handle anything? Didn't we believe that positive thinking could cure all ills, and that there wasn't anything we wouldn't be able to overcome if we just had the right attitude? And is it this way of thinking that may be making it even more difficult for us to see our parents starting to fail now?

If there is one thing we learned, it is that we don't have to suffer alone. Many of us have been to encounter groups, self-help groups or formal counselling. Some have been to psychiatrists. We're not afraid to ask for help, and we know it's easily available.

But our parents were raised in a different world. On the whole they were taught to suffer in silence, to grin and bear it. Most people feel that this may be part of the reason it's harder for them to accept the emotional aspects of the situation once they start having physical and mental troubles.

My father almost had a complete emotional breakdown before he went to talk with a counsellor, and I don't know if he would have gone if my mother's doctor had not insisted. If I had been there, I could have seen how much he needed help, but I was only able to visit three times in the six months before mom died. He seemed to be handling things fine when I did and when we talked on the phone, he said everything was okay.

What did the counsellor tell him? She told him not to spend ten hours a day in the nursing home staring at my mother. She told him he had to take care of himself and his own needs, or he would become a patient, too. She told him, basically, that he was alive, and that life for the living had to go on.

Would he have made it through the ordeal without this good advice? I don't know. But fortunately he accepted what the counsellor said and immediately made changes in his routine. He started visiting mother only two hours a day, and resumed some of his former activities, including seeing his relatives more often. He started cleaning house, taking care of the yard, and cooking.

If your parents don't want to share what they're feeling with you, and you don't want to pry and prod, what can you do? Many professionals feel that no matter how well someone seems to be handling things, he or she could still benefit greatly from a talk with a counsellor. You may have to make the appointment for your parent and drive him there, but try to make sure he goes before things reach the point where he may not be able to cope.

Pam Dawson, a clinical-nursing specialist in gerontology at the Sunnybrook Health Science Centre, told me that when a couple has been together for a long time, one partner's entering a care facility is a major disruption. All of a sudden, others are part of the relationship. Many people need counselling to deal with this intrusion.

Marilyn McGregor, an occupational therapist with Community Therapy Services in Winnipeg, adds: "Residents who have the most difficulty are those who always said they never wanted to go into one of those places, and so have negative perceptions even before they go in. But some residents vastly improve in a care facility because of better nutrition, stimulation, and so on.

"Some communities now have day programs which are usually held at the facility, and this is a helpful transition.

Marlien McKay says that the main problem for people who must adapt to a care situation is loss—of roles, options and control—and of choice, because it is often a crisis situation so there is no time to work through the stages. She offers the following advice:

"Plan ahead. Make small changes gradually. This is why facilities that offer levels of care are so excellent.

"Ease the transition, and thereby decrease your feelings of guilt. Contemplate the range of options of care (choice).

"Consider the individual's sense of loss, and encourage situations and opportunities that alleviate the feeling. This requires creative effort. For example, contrive with previous activities or clubs, such as bingo with friends from the old neighbourhood, meetings. Adjust old interests to adapt to the new environment. If she had a big garden, at least set up a window box of herbs. Bring familiar objects such as bedspreads, pictures and furniture. Encourage maintaining self-care activities, because function and ability preserve identity and dignity. Encourage participation in new activities."

Individuals who are mourning losses in their lives must have acknowledgement that these feelings are understandable. Care givers can gradually redirect these feelings by encouraging him to maintain or re-establish a routine and activities. Start with short-term, concrete, achievable steps. For example, if father always had a big garden, but has no interest after his stroke, encourage him to plant and care for some patio tomatoes. Encourage productivity by asking for their assistance with projects such as sorting old family photos. Encourage reminiscences by talking about the past.

Lorna Reimer adds: "Guilt is common among people who have cared for a relative at home, but can no longer handle it. Involving these family members with some aspect of the resident's care and keeping an open door for communication are important. Giving positive feedback and reminders on what they have done for the resident, and what they can still do, are also helpful.

"For people who are grieving the loss of their independence, I try to help them find something they can do, or find an alternate way to do a task, if it was really important to them. Discussing with them their worth as a person and the abilities they still have, even though they cannot do some things, helps to realign their thinking. But most important is to continue to treat them as a totally worthwhile person— spending time talking with them, smiling at them, asking them questions, asking what they like or don't like, and just being a friend."

To sum up . . .

- People accept care when they are young, as this is the natural course of things. But when they have been independent for a long time, having to accept care again can be a traumatic experience.

- If you see that your relative or another member of the family is taking things particularly hard, don't wait to call in a counsellor or social worker for a talk.

- Above all, be a friend. Be someone that people can talk to.

CHAPTER 7

WHAT TO LOOK FOR WHEN SHOPPING FOR A CARE FACILITY

I f you have the luxury of time, you can spend weeks or even months looking at care facilities before deciding which ones to make application to. You'll be able to check into dozens if you have time. Then you can select three or four favourites, and take your loved one to those so that she can make the final decision—unless, of course, she wants to go with you to see every one, but this can be very tiring.

If you must make a rush decision because of a medical emergency, then you may be able to look at only three or four before you have to choose—and the final decision will probably rest with the family, not with the person who will be moving into the facility.

But whichever way you go, there are some vital points you should keep in mind during your search. When you visit the first couple of facilities, you won't even know which questions to ask, but after you've seen a few, you'll know. You'll be able to see all kinds of differences. And that's precisely why you should try to visit as many as possible before you make any decisions.

David Wright, executive director of the Visiting Homemakers Association of Metropolitan Toronto, feels that you should approach this decision the way you would shop for a new home or a new car. You should consider yourself a consumer, and consumers have certain rights. Remember that even if you are not paying directly for the care facility, you are still paying. You should seek to get your money's worth in every area, and you have the right to choose based on consumer values. And if things don't seem entirely right, either before or after your mom moves in, you have the right to complain as a consumer.

If this sounds alien to you, it shouldn't. Mr. Wright points out that people used to believe they couldn't do anything about cars that turned out to be lemons. Who would try to fight the big car companies? Well, Ralph Nader told the people they could start banding together as informed consumers. They did, and they got action.

It's the same with care facilities. If enough people share the same concerns—when they go shopping for a room or after mom moves in—

eventually things will change. The government can't be any harder to deal with than those big car companies!

The book covering all aspects of the different types of care facilities in the different provinces is bigger than this book you're holding. It will be difficult working through the maze yourself, so you'll definitely want some help. Social workers and discharge planners in hospitals are probably the best people to start with. They will understand what is available in your area, and can tell you which facilities would be best for your mom's needs.

Ontario Nursing Home Association president Harvey Nightingale suggests you get a list of all the appropriate facilities within perhaps a half-hour drive from your home—the more convenient the location, the more you'll visit. Call the administrators of those places and make an appointment for a visit. But don't just take the formal guided tour. Walk through by yourself. Talk with residents, talk with the staff. After you've narrowed your choices, go back a few times to the ones that have made the final cut. Go once in the morning, make another trip in the afternoon, and again in the evening.

The first time you enter a nursing home, you may be shocked at the sight of so many old and frail people. Just remember that a nursing home is for people who are very old, but more importantly, very ill. People who cannot cope with the aspects of daily living without assistance. That's why they're there.

"Seeing frail elderly people en masse can be quite a shock, so be prepared," says Susan M. Ellis. "You'll see people asleep in chairs, heads back, mouths open. You'll see the cognitively impaired wandering around aimlessly. Residents may be wearing mismatched shoes or clothes inside out. These sights must not be assumed to be a reflection of the care these people are receiving.

"No institution can provide the one-on-one personal care that families can. Placement in a facility is usually necessary because family members are unable to take proper care of the senior. A facility has a professional team to do so.

"When family members burn out from performing these tasks, they have no energy to provide quality time to their loved one anymore. So let the professionals take over these jobs, and keep your energy for quiet walks, teas, reminiscing, touching and loving."

Making the choice

"When someone is moving from her own home into a care facility, you should take your time looking for one," Patricia Fleming told me, "because it's important to make the right choice the first time. Moving a second time can be more traumatic.

"I suggest that the families make up two lists—a list of what mom must have in her new home, and a list of what she would like to have. Try to make the 'must have' list as short as possible. Be flexible.

"The family can visit several places and see which facilities meet most of mom's wants and needs. When you've narrowed the list down to three or four places, take mom to see them. Write down how each one fits into the 'must haves' and the 'wants.' Then you can sit together and go over the list and, supported by the family, mom can make the final decision. If she has made the decision herself, she has a bigger stake in making it work, and this makes all the difference in the world. The more you're prepared, the more you know about the decisions, and the more information and thinking that's gone into it, the better it's going to be.

"If someone is alone, without family, the process would be the same. But she would have to depend on a volunteer escort service or transportation to visit several places. This might take time."

I spoke with Roma Maconachie, assistant director of occupational therapy, and Janice Cadogan, occupational therapy education coordinator, of Community Therapy Services in Winnipeg. They also feel that making this decision right the first time is very important.

They suggest that you look at the physical environment at the facilities and take into consideration what your loved one's current needs are. Let's say it's your mom, and she has arthritis and is confined to a wheelchair. How accessible are the various areas of the facility? Will she be able to get into the crafts room and the atrium? Or is there just one big room where all the people in wheelchairs spend all their time watching TV?

They also recommend that you ask every facility about their policy regarding residents who start to deteriorate either physically or mentally. Would mom have to move into a different wing or a different floor? If so, will she still be able to visit and maintain friendships with both the staff and other residents from the previous wing or floor? How would this be handled?

You'll also want to look into the various activity programs offered. How compatible are they to what mom likes to do and what she's interested in? Does everybody just sit around and watch TV all day every day?

Perhaps she's very physically disabled but she gets a lot of joy from looking at nature. Is there a garden she could easily get to? If she has Alzheimer's disease and wanders, is there a safe area where she can wander without being unduly restrained or agitated?

In other words, you should look at your loved one and at how the various facilities could meet her needs today and the potential needs of tomorrow.

If you know someone who already lives in a facility, he will be the very best source of information. He will know exactly how the actual day-to-day care is given, and how well it meets the residents' and their families' needs. He'll also be able to fill you in on staff attitude, which can really make the difference between a great place and a miserable place.

If you're hesitant to have your mom move into a smaller rural home and feel that a larger facility may be better, occupational therapist Lois Klassen from Community Therapy Services in Winnipeg offers this list of advantages and disadvantages of small rural homes.

Advantages

- close-knit relationships between staff and clients
- easy to communicate to staff information about client's special needs
- chance to get to know activity worker well; time for one-on-one contact
- easy access to outdoors; fields and parks nearby, birds, little traffic
- the town gets to know who the "wanderers" are and where they belong
- smoother transition into home because of home's close contact with community and hospital resources
- elderly from the community and churches often volunteer in the homes and become familiar with them before their loved ones or themselves move in

Disadvantages

- hard to avoid personality clashes
- low turnover of staff can mean that poor staff don't change or leave quickly
- sometimes there isn't funding for full-time activity staff because of small size of facility
- transportation around town may be difficult because of gravel roads, few paved ramps, sidewalks, and so on
- staff may not be as well educated as those in large cities; less opportunities for upgrading their training, and so on
- less access to special medical services—speech therapy, occupational therapy, orthotics, ophthalmology, dental services, and so on—might require a long ride in an ambulance; for example, to get a CAT scan or new glasses

Marilyn McGregor told me that she has come across a number of seniors who have gone back to the small towns where they were born when they needed a care facility, rather than staying in Winnipeg where their family members were. They thought they would know more people in their old home town. This usually turned out to be a mistake, and these seniors have few if any visitors. In her experience, staying close to the family works better—wherever the family is.

Specifics to look for

There are literally a hundred different things you could look into before choosing a care facility. Some are very important to your loved one who will be moving there, and others aren't. The following information comes from several people, and will give you a rough idea of some things you should look for.

Concerned Friends of Ontario Citizens in Care Facilities has developed the most comprehensive list of questions I've come across, with a method for scoring each facility you check out. To get a copy, send one dollar and a request for the Nursing Home Checklist to Concerned Friends, Box 1054, Station Q, Toronto, Ontario M4T 2P2.

- Is the facility convenient for visiting? Is there easy public transportation? If a facility is right on your way home from work, you'll stop a lot more often. If it's a real pain to get to, you'll find a lot of excuses not to visit very often. Many of your relative's friends may be old and unable to drive. They may be encouraged to visit more often if public transportation stops close to the facility.

- Is the facility close to a hospital? If a medical emergency happens, will it be easy to transport your relative to a hospital that can handle it or will it mean a two-hour ambulance ride?

- Is the building safe? Are there smoke detectors and a sprinkler system? Are exits clearly marked and well lit? Do you see emergency doors chained closed? If you're unsure about the fire safety, you can ask to see a fire safety inspection report. You should also be able to see a safety evacuation plan.

- Is the facility well lit throughout, or are there dark and dreary areas? Do desks and tables have sharp edges, which people may bump into? Are there handrails in all the hallways and grab bars in the bathrooms and by the beds? Do you see any obvious hazards to people who may not be able to get around too well, such as loose rugs or things stacked on the hallway floor? Is the furniture in the lounges and visiting areas heavy, so that it won't tip over?

- Is the decor cheerful and stimulating? Do you see a lot of bright colours, posters and plants? Or are the walls grey and unadorned? If there's something to look at in the halls, people may be more willing to leave their rooms for a walk. And besides, plain grey can be depressing. The facility should resemble a home as much as possible.

- Is there a garden or terrace with chairs or benches so that ambulatory residents can go outside on a nice day? Is there a ramp so that those in a wheelchair can also get out easily? How about a little flower bed or window boxes, not only for the beauty of nature, but also so that those who wish can putter in some real dirt?

- What activities are available? Ask to see the activities rooms. Do they look perfectly clean, as if nobody ever uses them, or are they full of happy people doing all sorts of things? How many activities people are there, and how regularly are they available? If people can only use the activities rooms and projects when they are supervised, you want the activities person to be there more than once a week.

- Are the bedrooms large enough to give people room to move? Is there plenty of space to manoeuvre a wheelchair or walker? Is there enough room so that people can bring a few personal things from home? Will it be easy to get in and out of bed?

- Is there adequate closet and drawer space? Is the furniture comfortable? Is there plenty of light for reading, including reading in bed? (If not, you can always bring a small clip-on light to put on the bed.) Are there some means available—curtains or screens—so that residents can have some privacy?

- Are the bathroom facilities close to the bedroom? Do they have plenty of room for a wheelchair or walker, or room enough so that two people can assist the resident while standing on either side of him? Are there grab bars and nurse call bells in the bathroom, and nonskid surfaces in shower stalls and bathtubs? How is the lighting?

Marlien McKay lists some of the things she would look for: a flexible, open-door visiting policy; guests welcome to bring children and pets; transportation available to take residents out on day trips; a "homey" atmosphere; residents encouraged to bring their own pictures, plants, a favourite chair; planned outings and activities; areas for residents to develop or maintain their skills, such as kitchens, gardens and woodworking shops; flexibility in the schedule, instead of rigidity.

Dr. Duncan Robertson also has some tips for selecting a good long-term care facility: location is important, because if it's too far away or in an inaccessible part of town, you'll visit less; a quick tour of a facility will tell you a lot about whether it is an environment in which you or a loved one can be cared for; ask the director of care or the administrator about policies, and see if they have an information brochure that describes some of the services that are available; be sure to ask some questions about medical care, such as whether the patient's own physician can continue to provide care there, or if there is a house doctor.

Some individuals will feel more comfortable in a place that specializes in the care of a particular ethnic or religious group. For others, proximity to services outside the nursing home are important.

If there is a residents' council or a group of relatives of the residents, and if you can access these groups, you might get some good inside information about the reputation of the facility, and the way in which it meets the needs of current residents.

Special considerations for people with Alzheimer's disease
If your dad is suffering from Alzheimer's or any other cognitive impairment, what you look for in a home may be slightly different. You should discuss the disease with your dad's doctor, someone who knows his case well, and ask how the doctor thinks it may progress. The disease moves very slowly in some people, and in others it gets very bad very quickly. Making the correct placement is even more important for people with diseases like these, as they need familiarity to feel secure. Having to move someone who is getting worse could be a terrible shock.

Some facilities have special units or floors prepared for people with Alzheimer's and similar diseases. I asked Dr. M. Oluwafemi Agbayewa, associate professor and head of the Department of Psychiatry, Prince George Regional Hospital, B.C., about them. "The word 'special' implies that special treatment will be provided," he says, "but unfortunately many so-called special-care units do not currently have the expertise or the staffing to provide what Alzheimer's or cognitively impaired patients need. If that is the case, then these units become just solitary units. But the goal should be to provide the specialized care that is needed, not just to keep these people away from the people who are not cognitively impaired.

"When we talk about older people in long-term-care facilities we generally ignore the fact that functioning is the basis of admission into facilities. In other words, if I have Alzheimer's disease but am still able to function well, like the majority of people in the early to middle stages of Alzheimer's, I shouldn't be put in one of these special-care units just because of the diagnosis. Whether someone goes into such a unit should be dependent on functioning—how well he gets along."

Dr. Nathan Herrmann, staff psychiatrist at Sunnybrook Medical Centre and an assistant professor at the University of Toronto, told me that there are some facilities that do not want to accept people with behavioural disturbances. To find this out, you should visit the facility and speak with the person doing the assessments, usually a social worker or a nurse. Ask what the criteria are for admission, and ascertain if your mom meets those criteria.

There are reasons for this. Dr. Herrmann said that he has seen disasters resulting from people who are very cognitively impaired being placed on floors for mildly impaired people, and vice versa. "Goodness of fit" is how he describes the ideal situation. And since family members are not always objective—or honest—in their assessment of their loved one's level of functioning, they do need an objective opinion. Situations where the family makes mom seem better or worse than she really is could result in these mismatches, and a lot of problems.

Making applications

The problem of not enough beds gets even more serious as more people are aging. And this won't change until services to help people stay in their homes longer are greatly increased. But even when they are, there will always be people who just cannot be kept at home. Anyone who thinks we'll be able to close all the care facilities once home care becomes adequate is dreaming. Too many people have no family to help them, and too many families cannot handle this difficult job.

And so we have waiting lists in most areas of the country. And we also have a lot of beds in hospitals being taken up by people who cannot go home and who are waiting for a bed in a facility. The cost is tremendous.

When they have openings, many homes take people first from these hospitals to free up the beds. That means, of course, that the people on the regular waiting list have to wait even longer.

Sorele Urman, director of the central intake department at the Baycrest Centre for Geriatric Care and Sheila Smyth, a social worker there, feel that if there's an immediate need for a bed in a care facility, you should make applications to at least five or seven different places. The wait at any facility is usually six months to a year, or maybe longer, depending on where you live. And the lists at the nicest places may be as long as five years. You can ask a social worker or discharge planner to call once in a while on your behalf, to ask how the waiting list looks.

But they also suggest that you yourself make contact with somebody at the facilities mom most wants to go into. Try to find somebody you feel you can communicate with. Then you can keep in touch with her, calling regularly to remind her that you're still waiting, and that you want to get mom into that facility the most. There's a chance your contact will be flattered that her facility is your first choice, and maybe this will help your case.

If you absolutely cannot handle the stress of caring for someone, and respite care and other services are not enough to help you, you may have to take some drastic measures. Some people admit the relative to a hospital for any reason they can think of, and then hope the hospital will be able to find him a bed. Some people take their story to the newspapers. Some people call their MP.

If you're absolutely desperate, you should talk with a social worker, counsellor or discharge planner, who can help you decide what to do. You can also call or write the people in the resource list who are ultimately responsible for the care situation in each province.

If you're at the end of your rope, do something—quickly. Don't become a patient yourself.

To sum up . . .

- There are all kinds of care facilities across the country. Seek some advice about what kind you should be looking at.

- Get a list of all the appropriate facilities within a reasonable distance of your home and check out as many as you can. Once you've narrowed the list to three or four, take mom along with you if she's able, and let her make the final choice.

- Finding the best place the first time is important, because moving later is very traumatic.

- We will always have a shortage of beds, so you may have to make application to a dozen places in order to find mom a bed. Be prepared to wait perhaps a year or more.

- If you cannot find a bed for your loved one and are about at the end of your rope, you may have to do something drastic to save yourself. Don't wait until you become ill, too.

CHAPTER EIGHT

EASING THE MOVE

Once your loved one has made the decision to move into a care facility, there are many things that have to be taken care of. Making the move is never easy, but with emotional support and help from the family, most people do get through it without too much pain.

Because care facilities always have waiting lists, you may find you have three to six months, or even a year or more to get everything in order. This usually works out for the best, because it gives the whole family a chance to adapt to the new life mom or dad will be starting.

You'll want to talk with the bank manager and probably a lawyer about accounts and important papers. You may want to open a safety-deposit box for some of mom's things if you don't already have one.

Most people start getting ready for the move by going through their possessions, deciding what they will keep and what they will give away. If you have the chance to see a room exactly like the one your parent will be moving into, you can take measurements and check on storage space.

Some facilities will allow her to bring some of her own furniture, but most don't have room. Some will have generous closets and a nice big dresser, but others will have very little space. It's good to know ahead of time, before mom starts going through her things.

Most places will allow residents to bring such personal items as pictures for the wall and a few knick-knacks, even if space is really limited. Just be sure to check ahead of time what is allowed. It's very difficult for people to part with all of their favourite things at once, so try to make sure mom takes a few things that really mean a lot to her. Some examples: personal photographs, favourite books, a treasured painting or piece of needlework. Also a good idea are things like a radio with a cassette player and cassettes of her favourite music, a clock and a calendar.

Encourage her to take along some craft supplies, favourite games, or cards. It can get pretty boring watching TV all the time. The nursing home my mother was in had a beautiful knitted afghan on every single bed, made by people who didn't have anything else to do—men included. If your mom is still able to do any kind of craft or needlework, perhaps everyone can chip in to keep her stocked with the necessary supplies.

Although it may be particularly difficult for mom to part with her jewellery, it may be wise. Even the best facilities have problems with theft. And of course there's always the possibility that she might absent-mindedly misplace a treasured heirloom bracelet herself. But it's probably safe for her to keep a wedding band, and perhaps a pendant on a chain, as they usually won't be taken off.

If you keep her best jewellery at your house, you can bring it for her to wear during special events. Always have her all decked out whenever you take her out for dinner or a family occasion. And bring it along with you for her to wear during parties and special occasions at the home, too, when you're there to keep an eye on it. Then take it back with you when you leave. In this way, she can still enjoy it, but it won't be in any danger of getting lost or stolen.

If mom is mentally alert, you'll have to discuss all this with her before she moves, and let her make the decision. She will already be giving up a lot when she moves, and if she decides to take the risk and keep her favourite bracelet or her grandmother's earrings with her, you should support her.

Sifting through a lifetime of accumulated possessions can be an arduous and heart-wrenching job for most people. Someone who has saved matchbooks and other mementos from every special dinner with her husband for sixty years or more may find it very difficult indeed to part with these things. But it's important that she have the privacy and time to sort through her belongings, and to cry over them if she wants to. Don't rush her. She's sorting through a lifetime of memories.

She will be able to keep some things with her—but not everything. It becomes a matter of priorities. Even private rooms in the most deluxe facilities have limited space. And since most people will be sharing a room with one or even three other people, there will be even less space.

If you have a year to do this job, mom can spend perhaps the first six months going through everything slowly and deliberately, looking at every photograph and memento, and picking out only the most valuable. If she's been a "saver" all her life, even after this there will probably still be too many things to take into her new home. So then she will have another few months to go through everything again.

Most people want to give things they can't take with them to family and friends. If mom has her heart set on certain gifts for certain people, respect her wishes, even if you don't understand. You may have had your eye on her ruby ring for years, but if she wants to give it to a young girl from down the street who has been kind to her, she should be able to without any recriminations from you. You'll never know exactly what that girl means to her or has done for her.

The things that mom has no specific plans for can be divided up among family members who want them, or they can be sold at a garage sale to bring in a little money for mom to take with her to her new home.

Clothing and personal-care items

What clothing she should take depends upon storage space, her physical condition and how often the laundry will be done. She will generally need enough clothes and undergarments to last a week, as this is usually how often the laundry is done, if done, by the facility. If you'll be doing the laundry, perhaps only every two weeks, then adjust the amount of clothing accordingly.

Many facilities ask that female residents wear short simple day dresses or gowns, as this makes dressing and changing of diapers, if used, easier. It's more difficult if someone is wearing a jogging suit. But most men wear jogging suits, and that seems okay. They're easy to wash and comfortable. Ask someone if they prefer a certain type of clothing at the home your mom will be going to before you go through her clothes. You may have to buy all new things.

People who are in wheelchairs will need warm clothing, as well as lap blankets and sweaters or shawls. Those who cannot get out of bed will need appropriate clothing to keep them covered and warm. All residents should have a warm coat for wearing outside.

Mom will also need a good warm bathrobe, and something to sleep in if the home does not supply gowns. Obviously someone who is incontinent will need extra clothes, as clean clothes sometimes get soiled the minute they're put on. And some stains don't wash out.

Warm socks are a must, as older people may have poor circulation in their feet—and it seems like the floors are always chilly. She'll need several pairs, and they should be in light colours so that her name can be marked on the soles. Most residents wear tennis shoes, recommended because they have nonslip soles. They can also be washed.

Be sure to ask which personal-care items are needed. Some homes supply toothpaste, shampoo, hand lotion and so on, free, but some don't. Some supply these things, but at inflated prices. If your mom wants her own things, take just a small supply of each, and replenish them when you visit. There's no sense in taking five bars of soap at one time. Also include some personal items, such as your mom's favourite perfume. Remember, this is her new home, and she should have as many familiar things around her as possible.

If you've ever been in the hospital, you know how cold and even alien those rooms are. There are no personal things, nothing to spell out who you are as an individual. You mom's new room at the care facility will be the same, until she brings in her personal little touches. Try to help her make the place homey.

Patricia Fleming told me the story of one of her clients who decided that it would be a whole new life, a whole new start, when she moved into a care facility. She was going to do it right.

She didn't want to take any of her old furniture with her—she wanted all new things. She was going to be rooming with a lovely woman, so she wanted all new clothes to look her best. She took her time and carefully went through everything she owned, but got rid of almost everything before she moved.

Some people want to cling to almost everything they own, but this lady was different.

If you can help your loved one develop just a bit of this attitude, the move will be easier to handle.

Labelling and listing belongings

Absolutely everything that mom takes with her to the care facility should be carefully labelled. You can buy an indelible laundry marker to mark all the clothing, and certain permanent marking pens will write on everything else, even glass. Mark everything with her last name and room number. And that includes the pictures on the wall.

My father carefully marked my mother's name on the care labels of each piece of her clothing, but things disappeared anyway. He found a sweater in the TV room that was identical to hers once, but he couldn't prove anything because the label had been cut off, and the name with it. So from then on, when he bought her anything new, he took it to a friend who ran a trophy and sports-patch company. This man used his specialized equipment to thickly embroider her name and room number in a conspicuous place right on the front of every garment and canvas shoe. Nothing ever disappeared again. You may have to resort to similar actions.

In other words, don't be afraid to boldly label things if theft is a problem at the place mom moves into. Nobody would steal a walker that had SEYMOUR emblazoned in bright red permanent tape on the side. Just explain to mom why you may have to mark up some of her things, or why her clothes may have to have her name and room number in a place everyone can see. She will probably agree that it's better than losing them forever.

You should also make a list of absolutely everything your loved one is bringing with her when she comes into the home. List the titles of the books, describe the pictures on the wall. Describe clothing in detail, including colour, pattern and size. Then if something gets lost in the laundry, it can be reunited with the rightful owner. Keep a copy of this list and give one to the staff when mom is admitted. It should be kept in her personal file.

In addition to clothing and other personal effects, don't forget to list and label things like eyeglasses, dentures and hearing aids. These things are easily lost or misplaced. Glasses and hearing aids can be permanently etched with the resident's name if you take them to the place where you bought them. Dentures should have been marked with her name at the time of manufacture, but if they weren't, this can be done anytime. Just ask your dentist.

If you bring anything like a clock or cassette player, record the serial numbers as well as the model and make. Mark cassette tapes with a permanent marker, not just with something like a piece of tape that can be easily removed.

Although care facilities do not take responsibility for missing or damaged things, this list will help them keep track of a resident's belongings.

Of course every disappearance is definitely not a theft. Sometimes residents lose their own things. Laundry workers are always finding dentures, glasses and hearing aids in the folds of sheets or pockets of robes. All kinds of things are left in activities rooms and at the nurses stations.

And all care facilities have a few residents who wander about aimlessly and who occasionally pick up things in their wanderings. These things generally turn up somehow, somewhere. But the staff will not be able to return them to their owners if they are not marked in some way. So even if mom goes into a place where everyone will tell you there is no theft, it's still wise to mark everything.

How to minimize the disappearance of your loved one's possessions[1]

Permanent disappearance of residents' clothes and other personal possessions is a common complaint. It is a serious issue because it affects the residents' quality of life, it violates the Bill of Rights, it strains the families' financial resources, and stealing is a criminal offence. Here's what you can do:

1. Make two copies of a list of all her belongings. Take them to the administrator to sign. Leave one copy for her file and keep the other one.

2. Label clothing with indelible ink or sewn-in commercial name tapes.

3. Have her name etched into dentures, glasses, hearing aids, walkers, canes and wheelchairs.

4. Never leave large amounts of cash with her. If she can manage money, advise her to keep only small amounts. Otherwise, arrange for an account with the tuck-shop.

5. When you buy articles, keep and copy the receipts. Show these and the items to the administrator, ask for the receipts to be signed and the copy

---

[1] Reprinted with permission from the Concerned Friends of Ontario Citizens in Care Facilities newsletter, spring 1988.

to be filed. Keep the original. Show the items to the charge nurse and other staff members on the floor.

6. Each time you visit, check to make sure that everything is there.

When items have disappeared
1. Ask the charge nurse and staff. If you are told that the item was "lost in the laundry" or that "a wandering resident has walked off with it," request that the item be located.

2. Inform the administrator and/or the director of nursing and request that items be found within a specified time limit—one or two days— and follow up with a letter.

3. If the time limit has passed and the items have not been found, consider them stolen and report to the local police and to your provincial nursing-home authority. Request them to investigate and to report to you in writing. Follow up with a written request.

It is often assumed that, because elderly people live in institutions, that the law doesn't apply to them. That is not true. Their address changes, but they retain the same rights and responsibilities as any Canadian, including protection under the law. Because stealing is a criminal offence, the police should be called in to investigate.

The Bill of Rights states: "Every resident has the right to keep in his or her room and display personal possessions, pictures and furnishings in keeping with safety requirements and other residents' rights." And: "Every resident has the right to live in a safe and clean environment." If possessions are taken, these rights are violated and the provincial nursing home authorities must be told. See the resource list in the back of the book for addresses.

The loss of dentures, glasses and hearing aids diminishes the quality of a resident's life and health. Loss of dentures obviously diminishes nutrition. Loss of glasses and hearing aids deprives a resident of the ability to communicate. These appliances are all expensive to replace.

Losing one's cherished possessions is a traumatic experience for anyone. And how much more so for residents who have so little.

Moving day
The day your loved one moves to his new home will probably be greeted with a mixture of anticipation and anxiety. And probably a few tears on both sides. But if it has been dad's decision to make this move, you may even find that he's been looking forward to starting his new life, almost the way a young person looks forward to going off to university for the first time. Remember, although he will be giving up parts of his old life, he will also be gaining a whole new life—new friends and new activi-

ties. Especially if recently he's been home alone a lot, this new change will be quite an adventure.

Plan to spend a few hours at the care facility with him, helping him unpack and settle in. Then if he's feeling up to it, you may want to go around with a nurse who will show both of you the crafts and recreational rooms, the cafeteria and tuck-shop, and so on.

Introduce yourself and your dad to as many people as you can. This is his new home now, so you'll want to get to know all the neighbours. Try to be positive about the experience, even if your heart is breaking. Your dad will be able to feel your vibes, and it may upset him if you're anxious.

Stay with him through at least the first meal. He may then want to take a nap, so that's a good time to leave. Visit frequently in the first few weeks—every day if possible. If you can't make it every day, try to line up family members and friends so that someone will show up. The adjustment may be difficult, and at the beginning he'll want to see a familiar face or two every day.

If the move wasn't a choice

Some people who end up in care facilities have had no choice. Many admissions to facilities are made directly from hospitals. Perhaps your dad has had a stroke, or grandma has fallen and badly injured herself, and it's the doctor's opinion that he or she will never be able to return home.

And sometimes people get so impaired because of Alzheimer's or other cognitive problems that they just aren't aware of what is going on. There is no way they could have helped make a choice concerning their care. When the time comes that they cannot stay at home, they will have to be moved into a care facility.

In a case where dad is still functioning mentally, you can and should consult with him regarding the move, even if there's no choice. Ask him which clothes he wants, which books, which pictures for the wall. He won't have the opportunity to go through his possessions and select what he wants, so you'll have to handle this. Don't rush him. Treat the task with love, respect and sensitivity.

Even if your loved one is so impaired that the doctors feel he doesn't know at all what's going on, you still owe it to him to make the move as pleasant as possible. Put yourself in his place. You know what colour shirts he likes best, and which plants and pictures he's fond of. Select these favourite things for his room. Then if he does have lucid moments along the way, he won't feel as if he's in a totally alien environment. He'll be surrounded by familiar possessions.

Doctors are not sure if seriously impaired people do have these flashes of lucidity, but it is a possibility. Even when my mother was almost in a coma, she would still stare at me sometimes, like she was really aware of what was happening, but just couldn't communicate. You never know.

To sum up . . .

- Even if your parent has decided to move into a care facility, adjustment may be difficult. Give mom or dad plenty of time to think, and if necessary, cry.

- All care facilities will allow a few personal things, but how many depends on how much room is available. Try to check out a similar room before your parent starts going through her possessions, so she will know ahead of time how much she can keep.

- Allow her the total freedom to do what she wishes with her lifetime of possessions and memories.

- Theft is a problem in some care facilities. Label everything and make a thorough list. If anything disappears, make a fuss about it. Mom has had to give up most of her possessions, so she should be able to keep the few remaining things without fear of their being stolen.

- If a parent is admitted to a care facility without a choice, you owe it to him to carefully go through his possessions and bring him what you know he would like to have. Put yourself in his place.

CHAPTER NINE

CARE THAT MAKES LIFE WORTH LIVING

People have a better quality of life, feel happier, and are probably healthier if they remain as physically and mentally active as they can. Obviously the degree to which people are able to remain engaged in life varies a great deal. But even people with disabilities or limitations can still have a spark in their eye, and an interest in the people around them and their surroundings. They can still contribute something to their environment, and this is important to quality of life. People, I believe, need to feel that they are contributing something—advice, warmth, comfort, humour, ideas—in order to have a meaningful life.

Older people, women especially, have a need to comfort and nurture. They have always done this, and even now when they might not be able to take care of themselves completely, they still have a desire to continue helping others. So if you can find some way for them to make a real contribution, you'll be soothing their spirits in wonderful ways.

I have already mentioned how older women who can still handle a crochet hook can make beautiful scarves or afghans to give as gifts to family members and friends. All you have to do is make sure they don't run out of yarn. Elderly people who cannot do this sort of thing could perhaps dictate old family recipes or even tell great stories about the family history. (If someone wants to do this, be sure to tape the stories for future generations.) Or you could bring in the old photos and have mom tell you who all those strange people are. Dad could tell the grandkids how to catch fish.

In other words, it doesn't take much to make people feel valued. It just takes a little creativity, a little thought, and you'll be able to come up with something that will make your mom or dad feel special.

Some care-facility residents may come to feel their lives have little value because many choices have been taken away from them. Now they have to fit into the routine of an institution. A person who has always taken a shower every day may now get one only every third day, because that's when everyone is showered or bathed. People who normally stay up late and sleep in may have trouble doing so, and may have to adjust their schedules to the facility's routine. The same applies to meals, which are generally always at the same time.

So herein the problem. On the one hand, everyone says you need to allow people to make choices to keep them independent and to help them live with dignity. But on the other hand, so many choices are disallowed. If your dad moves into a care facility and wants to watch TV until three in the morning, just see how long that will be permitted.

"For many people who go into care facilities, the environment and the resources do not permit them to feel a sense of continuity from their previous lives, nor a sense of being at home," says Pam Dawson. "The focus within care facilities is often providing care rather than enabling people to continue to live as adults and to have normal experiences."

Some choices *can* be accommodated. This will be more likely to happen in a smaller home rather than a larger one, where consistent routine is more important. So if you know your dad can't fall asleep until three in the morning, and likes to watch TV or read most of the time, you can try to find him a place where he can have a private room. Then he can stay up as long as he wants, and won't disturb anybody. (Buy him a TV with earphones.) This is a far better solution than having him move into a very routine-driven facility where he might be obliged to take a strong sleeping pill every night so he can go to bed with everyone else at nine-thirty—or even earlier!

"It is easier for staff to cope with residents if the staff follows a rigid daily routine," Concerned Friends director Joan Fussell told me. "For instance, a person's preference to sleep in late and go to bed late may be impossible to accommodate in a facility that requires night staff to get people up very early in the morning to relieve the burden of work for the day staff. The residents may be given no choice nor respect in this manner.

"My suggestion is that people try to assert their preferences as much as they can to make it clear what they do and do not want within realistic options. Relatives can be a big help by reminding the staff of those preferences and insisting on their being respected. It may be hard for a relative to stand up for the resident, but it may be much harder for the resident to stand up for himself."

Harvey Nightingale explains that routines are generally set up because of cost. Take meals, for instance. You have to feed people at certain times because that's when there is adequate staff available for this purpose. Nursing homes generally try to have two choices on every menu for breakfast and dinner, and occasionally for lunch. There's a tray with juice and snacks in the afternoon, and fresh fruit in the evening.

If someone was unable to eat breakfast, the staff usually brings him something later. But the kitchens are cooking for a hundred or more people, so naturally they can't accommodate everybody all day long—as soon as they've cleaned up from breakfast, they have to start making lunch! They recognize that each resident is an individual, and that tastes will vary. They try to have enough variety in the menus so that there will be something everybody likes.

There are other things about institutions that have always bothered me. When I see movies or documentaries about care facilities and see people being talked to and treated like children, especially concerning activities, I cringe. For instance, they will line up all the people who are in wheelchairs and toss a ball back and forth while saying things like "That's a good boy!" when someone catches it. To me, this is just awful. I'm certain many of the residents did not want to participate in such degrading and childish activities, but if they'd refused to cooperate, they would have been made fun of.

I asked several people about situations like this, which I consider to be a real—and yet easily avoided—loss of dignity. I also asked about situations in which people do not want to go to bed or eat at the same times as everyone else.

"I think that the bottom line is that every person should be self-determining," responds Kathleen Gates. "Each person has the right and should be able to express his likes and dislikes. I really resent the schedules in some long-term care facilities. I think there should be more flexibility in terms of when meals are served, when people choose to have their bathing done, all kinds of things. We have to start looking at life patterns that people have had, values that people hold and what people choose to do with their time.

"I don't think people should be forced into groups if they've always been loners. What we have to do is look at people's pasts, and if they weren't gregarious in the past, they are not going to be that way in the present or the future.

"We have to look at past interests, abilities and social networks, and try to help people arrive at something that's best for them at the moment."

Patricia Fleming agrees. "The most important factor in a care facility is the staff attitude. This is something you can usually check out before you choose a facility—when you visit, just watch how the residents are treated.

"If they're treated like little girls and boys, then I would beware. I would also beware if people aren't spoken to at all.

"The big fear that people have when they go into any kind of institution is the fact that the doors are going to close and that's going to be it. They will be taken away from the real world forever. But it's important to make them feel they are still members of the real world, and one way to do this is to allow dignity and choices."

Some people choose, for various reasons—because they are tired, unwell, unwilling or unable to make necessary effort—to opt out, not relate, not contribute. And I believe they should have that right.

All that relatives and friends, or staff at a care facility can do is offer options, make people aware of the choices open to them, and support the choices each individual makes. But well-meaning types have to recognize that forcing people to participate in activities they have no interest in, or thinking they know what is best for another human being, is patronizing.

"Too many people fail to appreciate the individuality of residents and respect their individual needs," Ms. Fussell adds. "Residents are too often treated more as commodities than as real, living human beings deserving of love and kindness and respect."

Etta Ginsberg McEwan, director of social work at Baycrest Hospital in Toronto and author and lecturer on the treatment and understanding of families dealing with aged and ill relatives, says: "We know all the complaints about institutionalization. There's lack of privacy, nobody's going to get his or her own room. The government doesn't have that kind of money. But there are things that could be done.

"The institutions are too large. This kind of living is alien. This is not the way you grew up. You don't expect to be living in a huge building with so many roommates, where you don't choose your neighbours. Some people who are isolated, who have lost all their family, are fine in large institutions. For some people this kind of congregate meets a lot of needs.

"But I would think that, maybe in the future, institutions would be more or less smaller homes within the community, with real intensive nursing care. I don't mean group homes like foster care for the elderly in reasonably good health, but smaller places within the community. Some institutions are beautiful, but they're still set apart from the real world. You enter them and you enter the world of the old and the sick.

"You can't really help people adjust—you just help people cope. Life is a drag. You only live one minute at a time, and you try to do the best you can. It's when you're called upon to meet a crisis—and institutionalization is a crisis—that we call upon these coping skills. The people who don't cope well are those who probably didn't cope too well with crises when growing up.

"And you can't pretend to people—like, 'there, there, honey, it's okay.' I'd really hate that. But that goes on, and probably the most difficult thing is that when somebody comes into a care facility a lot of education is needed for staff. We put so much emphasis on helping the resident cope, but really how they cope will depend upon the attitude of the staff.

"The stuff you took for granted or the things you did in the privacy of your own home, we sit in judgement on. You get labelled uncooperative or manipulative, but meanwhile everybody's manipulating all day to survive in the world. So it's up to the staff, and I think that the staff needs a lot of help because staff attitudes and staff behaviour are not intentional and not purposeful; it's just that everyone is so frightened and feels so vulnerable that this might happen to her.

"To see the unhappiness in some people who have to come into the institution, it's really painful. It's hard to deal with.

"There are some things about institutional life—I mean, look at how the beds are. They don't have double beds. When you come into an institution it's already considered you are asexual, so you don't have double beds. That is just a symbol of all that goes on."

Ms. Fussell continues: "Family members can see that their loved one really is taken proper care of according to his wishes. First, the family should make those wishes clearly known, and repeat them. Second, one of the best assurances is to be at the facility to visit the relative as often as possible, and at different times of the day. Third, when care is not adequate, the family should keep notes, including details of dates, times, places, people present or people responsible, and what was said. Then they can speak to the supervisor or administrator."

But Susan M. Ellis feels that "families, instead of criticizing, would further the cause of satisfying individual needs by recruiting more volunteers and asking how they themselves could help out.

"A care plan is made up for each resident. Families and residents can be involved in updating those care plans. In many institutions, relative support groups and residents' councils provide opportunity to communicate and bring about change."

Marcia Wargon says that while the current alternatives in provision of care are not ideal, that's all there are. "Therefore, people need to be helped to express feelings about types of care and have some degree of real involvement in the provision of care, perhaps through a residents' or family council in the care facility. People should be encouraged to assert themselves in demanding and helping to develop the kind of care facilities they want for their relatives, through involvement in agencies, programming in facilities, and so on."

Dr. Duncan Robertson feels that even if an older person is disabled, it is important that he continue to do the things he is still capable of. "A person may have some degree of mental impairment, some degree of physical impairment, but his main interest in life is gardening and he wants to go out in the garden. But because of his confusion or because they're worried he may fall, family members may be concerned. They don't want him falling or injuring himself. So their reaction to this is to say, 'Well you shouldn't do anything like that at all, because of the risk of injury.'"

But that person may become more disabled in other aspects of life simply because he is not exercising anymore, not getting out, and has lost a major interest in life. Dr. Robertson calls this a "secondary disability."

The initial disability is the one caused by the physical or mental health problems, but the secondary disability is the one caused by the disuse of a faculty or some ability the senior is quite capable of exercising. And so often a secondary disability occurs from the best of intentions of a family trying to protect him from injury.

To stop this sort of thing, frail and dependent people should be not only allowed but encouraged to exercise all their remaining faculties to the fullest, and to tolerate and to accept reasonable risks.

"For example, one of the greatest risks in the frail elderly is the risk of falling and fracturing something," Dr. Robertson explains. "But there is absolutely no way you could completely eliminate these risks. The older person has impaired control of his body posture, and thus a much higher risk of falling for a number of reasons related both to aging and to the medical problems people get.

"When seniors do fall they have a much higher risk of serious injury, primarily fractures. But in order to minimize or eliminate injuries from falling, you'd have to put such severe restrictions on a person's life that life may not be worth living."

So, if we're worried about grandpa or dad, how can we allow him to choose what he wants to do, and then have the courage to let him go ahead and do it?

You should make reasonable modifications to the environment to make sure there aren't any serious hazards, such as loose rugs, and offer and make available reasonable appliances or aids, such as walkers or canes, to enable him to walk safely. And then it is important for the family and care givers to accept the risks inherent in his continuing to get around.

Falls can and do occur in long-term care facilities, in hospitals and in patients' homes. But Dr. Robertson feels it is important for families not to feel guilty or to blame themselves if a fall should occur after all reasonable steps have been taken to minimize the risk. He warns that excessive concern about protecting a frail, dependent relative from injury may sometimes lead to secondary disabilities.

As Evelyn Wexler explains, "Care facilities should attempt to, and should want to, create a living environment that capitalizes on people's abilities and invites family participation. They shouldn't be places that people feel they are coming to because they are losers, or because they can't manage anymore—or because nobody else wants them.

"You can create a living environment that's still going to be relevant to them, and still going to allow them to have quality of life. That is the biggest challenge. There is a tendency when you're working in a big facility to be too regimented, causing people to lose not only autonomy but individuality. That has to be monitored very carefully.

"I think we should look more at trying to plan care using the residents themselves if possible, or their families, and figure out care plans that will really be relevant to individuals.

"We might find, in fact, that sometimes we provide too much care. We tend sometimes to take too much away from people, to take over and provide everything."

The care facility must follow a schedule to accommodate the needs of so many individuals living in a communal setting. This translates into some loss of independence, some loss of choice.

The environment may not be as pleasant, or may not be what the care giver believes the resident would like or deserves, and sometimes those concerns get translated into an almost antagonistic stance toward the facility and to the staff who work there.

There have been some studies on the care giver's stress, and the anxiety and problems suffered by care givers of frail old people. These studies have looked at the level of their stress before their loved one is admitted into a long-term care facility and after. You might expect that when their loved one is admitted to a facility, that the care giver's stress would diminish. But in fact, findings of this study show that it doesn't decrease at all.

What people find when their loved ones are admitted to care facilities is that problems don't go away, they just change. The family members have to deal with feeling guilty and feeling that they were inadequate in providing care. Now the family members have to relate to new care givers who do things differently from the way they believe their loved one would prefer.

Obviously some of these problems can be relieved if family members communicate with the facility staff, but very often those who are providing direct care are very busy and have insufficient time to deal with the needs of the family, as well as the needs of the resident.

A lot of people live outside the big cities. Sometimes not having as many resources is helpful, because it calls on people to use their own creativity to give the care facilities a real homelike setting. Try to broaden the thinking so that you not only have the people who are involved in the direct care at the facility, but also other people, so that you're making connections between the community at large and the community that exists within that facility.

Pets should be brought in. Kids should be brought in to visit. It's so great when you see an older person and a child knitting together. Or there are foster-grandparent programs. There are a lot of kids today who don't have an older person in their lives, and this is a good way for them to learn the natural course of life. And they'll also learn all kinds of other fascinating things from seniors.

Of course it unfortunately happens sometimes that a staff shortage is so severe and existing staff is so overworked that they don't want to have to clean up after a group—it seems like too much trouble. Sometimes it's easier to sedate people and put them in the hallway. That's why education is so important. We need to talk about aging, because all of us need to grapple with it. We're all going to get old.

But no matter how much education any of us has experienced, we haven't been old yet. And if you haven't been old yet, you can't fully appreciate what it is to be old.

Lorna Reimer feels that, although moving into an institution may not be a first choice, it may be a necessary one if family or other resources are not adequate to meet all the care and social needs. "These are especially apparent when the family is nonexistent, unable or unwilling to care for the individual. Not all people are capable of caring for others, especially when it includes all the physical self-care needs. We need to consider that it's okay to place someone in a long-term care facility when other care options are insufficient, and take a positive approach to it.

"Even though someone moves into an institution, it should be considered the resident's home, and this change of attitude would make a big difference for staff and families. Generally persons in nursing homes are called residents, not patients, as 'patient' implies illness and implies that others have control.

"The resident and family should be part of the team and actively participate in determining the goals and specific routines of care. As the staff does not know the unique habits and traits of a new person moving in, the resident can benefit greatly if the family tells the staff who the resident is and was. Past history is very important, especially when memory impairment exists. Likewise, the staff can explain the routines and services of the facility, including the medical, personal care, therapeutic, recreational and other programs offered. The goals and needs of the resident can then best be met by combining the information from both to formulate an individual-care plan."

Social isolation is often a big concern of the elderly living at home, especially if they are living alone in a large or urban community. Unless someone has a strong network of friends and relatives, days may go by when he sees nobody but perhaps the Meals on Wheels volunteer. And many people worry about falling or having a heart attack when nobody is around to help them.

Nursing homes can offer not only medical and personal care, but provide easy access to other people for things like playing cards, games, doing group activities or just social visiting. Nobody is alone in a care facility unless he really wants to be.

Residents, of course, no longer have to take out the garbage, buy groceries, wash clothes or cook nutritious meals, and so do not have to worry about these daily activities, which are frequently a bigger concern to the family than their relative's medical problem.

Another positive aspect of most care facilities is the easy access to special medical care and therapy. Problems may be picked up sooner by the medical staff, or just because residents are being attended to daily. For example, a nursing attendant may identify early bowel or skin problems during routine baths and toilet assistance. Regular exercise and therapeutic treatment can often improve the resident's physical well-being. She may not have had the benefit of this at home because of a lack of services or difficulty getting to a service.

"Attitude is probably the most important word I can use to summarize what makes or breaks any situation," Ms. Reimer continues. "This is the same for staff and volunteers of long-term-care facilities as it is for the residents, and their families and friends. A positive or pleasant attitude goes a long way to create a homey environment, more so than the best-decorated facility or the one with state-of-the-art equipment.

"This is one thing I would recommend people put first on their list when checking out a facility: when and how often do the staff members smile? Are staff members—including dietary and housekeeping staff—talking to the residents, or do they just push them away or shove things like pills or food at them? What is the atmosphere like? Are residents sitting around in small groups, or are they all lined up in long rows merely watching the world go by? I am not sure if this is because some facilities have been designed with inadequate lounge space or if the residents have nothing else to do, or unknown reasons! Likewise the attitude of the resident and family helps create the atmosphere, whether positive or negative."

Patricia Fleming thinks it's the same for everybody—not just for the elderly, or for people in facilities. "So much depends on your attitude and your approach to where you are and your situation, no matter what it is. People who are open and friendly and try to make the best of a situation are going to get further ahead than those who are complaining and groaning and feeling sorry for themselves all the time. Life is always better for those who are cooperative."

Unfortunately, attitudes are not easy to change, especially if they have been ingrained for a lifetime. Ethnic and cultural background have a strong influence, as well.

Some residents seem to change completely the moment they walk through the door of a care facility. They may refuse to walk and demand a wheelchair. They may refuse to dress themselves. They might not even want to come out of their rooms for meals. Their attitude may be that they deserve a rest because they have worked hard all their lives—and many of them did as impoverished, immigrant farmers and labourers—and that the nurses are here to do everything for them. This "I'm sick, you take care of me" attitude needs to be changed throughout our society and especially in our health system.

Ms. Reimer told me about one positive example—Mrs. R., an elderly woman in a rural community with ALS (amyotrophic lateral sclerosis, or Lou Gehrig's disease). Mrs. R. had been widowed for about five years and was staying with her daughter prior to her admission into long-term care. Home care had provided regular assistance for medical monitoring and bathing, as well as rehabilitation to maintain function and mobility.

She was on oxygen, which was supplied and monitored, and had received a power wheelchair. Even though Mrs. R. was managing well with this wheelchair, could walk with a walker for short distances, and could dress and feed herself independently, she chose to be admitted to a long-term-care hospital. She could very likely have managed to stay at home for several more months with the support system available. Her choice was made to allow her family more independence, as her disease would inevitably make her increasingly more dependent on them for care. As this was her own choice, she has maintained a positive attitude and participates in life as much as she is able. Her family visits frequently, and she no longer worries about being a burden to them.

Ms. Reimer also told me the story of an elderly widow who was physically well but was unable to cope because of severe depression following her husband's death. Mrs. K. lived in a bungalow in a small city, and although she had home care—homemaking and nurse monitoring—she had no means of transportation, and no relatives or close friends for support. Her husband had been her closest friend, and her nearest relative lived several provinces away.

Volunteers and a church support group were contacted, and members paid friendly visits and assisted with shopping. After keeping Mrs. K. at home for a year and a half, a physician finally had to place her in a nursing home because her depression had created additional problems—poor nutrition and physical safety. For example, once she ran out into the street for help after a pot caught fire on her stove.

Independence can mean doing as much for yourself as you are able, or doing what you feel is most important if you do not have the physical stamina, because of fatigue or disease, to do everything. That means you may still get up and dress yourself, walk to breakfast, and then visit another resident or attend a morning news discussion group, but you don't have to make your bed or do the dishes or clean the tub.

"Change is always difficult and often more so as people become older," believes Marcia Wargon. "How to assist people in considering change requires a clear understanding of the individual, relationships within the family situation, the alternatives available, and the preferences of the person and his family.

"Counselling about the need for change, opportunities to become familiar with the alternative in a gradual way, being able to bring with one particularly significant items—all can ease the pain. Unfortunately, in some cases where the failing individual cannot comprehend or accept the need for change, the care givers may need support in making the change in a direct and unequivocal manner.

"This can be true for a care facility or for in-home help. It may be necessary for the care giver to leave when help comes in or to leave the person in a residence when he's taken there. Staff in the residence or in-home help must be trained to deal with the resistance, anger and fear of the individual, and the family must be supported through the period of adjustment. How well staff can handle these difficult situations varies depending on training and agency policies.

"There are no easy answers. Helping aging individuals and their families through this later period of life requires sufficient well-trained staff in all helping agencies and facilities. The implications for society as a whole in providing people and places that we could all feel satisfied with is another area to be considered."

It basically boils down to what Dr. John B. Bond, associate professor of family studies at the University of Manitoba told me. "People must create environmental, financial, home and institutional settings that they would like for their parents, and ultimately for themselves." If this is kept in mind, everyone will be happier.

Please don't forget the staff

Never forget that it is the staff in a care facility who makes the difference between the residents' having enriching and valuable lives or a boring existence.

Everyone I spoke with feels that people who work in long-term-care facilities are angels. And there are never enough of them. The work is often dirty and difficult, the hours are long, there's seldom a chance to sit down, the benefits are sometimes scanty, and the pay is far too low. And on top of that, they are always being criticized!

But if the work is so difficult and the pay so low, how can more people be brought into this type of work? As more people age, we will need even more nurses, more aides, more cooks and cleaners in care facilities.

Working with the elderly and sick is hardly a piece of cake. Many older people are not "beautiful," the way children are. People who don't feel well are often chronic complainers and if someone has been an unhappy person all her life, she certainly won't change when she's older.

So higher pay alone won't be enough to draw people into this line of work; people who go in it just for the money won't last long. It takes a very special, caring human being to work in a care facility. Someone whose heart is much bigger than the callouses on her feet after she's worked a few double shifts in a row.

Most people feel that what is needed is a real appreciation for those who do this difficult work. They need to be valued for the care and love they give, and valued for being there when nobody else can or wants to be.

"A good administrator will promote staff esteem and control, and this improves the care that seniors receive," says Bernard Bouchard, administrator of the Bourget Nursing Home in Bourget, Ontario.

Sure, like every one of us, angels also have bad days. It can be pretty nerve-wracking trying to care for far too many residents when three aides are off sick and there just aren't enough hours in the day to get everything done. It can also be frustrating trying to do so many things for people on such a strict budget.

So if occasionally a person taking care of your loved one snaps at you, please try to understand. And if everything isn't always done to your satisfaction, don't be too quick to blame the staff. Sometimes there are no options. Unfortunately, budget and time constraints govern too much of what goes on in facilities these days.

If you really want to change things, lobby your MP for better salaries, as this will attract more people into the profession. More staff means that more can be done for residents. Lobby for more money for the homes, as this will improve everything from the food to the state of the paint on the walls. Lobby for more recognition of the difficult work these people do day in and day out.

Above all, value and appreciate the care that is given your loved one. When something goes right, say something. When mom has her hair done and looks great, say something. When dad raves about his great afternoon in the patio garden, find out who took him out there and thank her.

When my father visited my mother, he constantly called the nurses and aides Florence. Of course, they always replied, "My name's not Florence!"

But his explanation always brought a big smile to their faces. "You sure look like Florence Nightingale to me!" It was a simple way of conveying the appreciation he felt.

"I think that if everybody started valuing the staff more it would be excellent for everyone," Kay Jacobson, program development director of the Visiting Homemakers Association of Toronto, told me. "I know from my own experience that thanks goes a long way.

"A written thank-you or a phone call is truly treasured. In fact, the people who work in facilities generally get so few thank-you notes that when they do get one, they put it on the bulletin board.

"We all need to be stroked. We need to be told we gave great service. It's so easy to say thank-you. But don't stop there. Also send a letter to the facility's administrator, the newspaper, and even to your MP, praising the great care your loved one is getting."

My father also used to bring in goodies to show his appreciation to the people taking care of my mother. Staff members were forbidden to accept gifts like money, so he'd regularly bring in a box of candy or a cake or cookies from a bakery.

Of course he got to know the nurses and aides who were on duty when he visited, and he never saw the ones on the night shift. But he left tokens of appreciation for all of them.

Gifts like his are certainly appreciated, but a thank-you note goes a long way, too.

To sum up . . .

- People should be encouraged to stay engaged in life. No matter how old or sick they are, they can still do things, still make choices. Don't take this away from them.

- There are many things you can do to help ensure that your loved one receives care that makes life worth living. Don't assume that just because she's in a facility now your obligation has ended.

- Understand that everything cannot always be done for your loved one to your personal standards. There are not enough hands and not enough hours in the day. If you think care is really lacking, why not pitch in and help?

- Never forget that it's the staff who ultimately determine how your loved one will live. Show them that you appreciate them, and you and your loved one will be treasured in return.

CHAPTER TEN

THE IMPORTANCE OF VISITING

One of the main reasons people fear moving into a care facility is that they will be abandoned. No matter what someone's physical or mental state, nurses will tell you that she will watch at the window with tears in her eyes as the family leaves after dropping her off. Even if she wanted to move into the facility and was looking forward to it, nothing is sadder than watching loved ones drive away that first time, and wondering if you'll ever see them again.

In most families, children are not separated from parents until they go off perhaps to college or university the first time. But when that happens, at least the parents know the children will be back for holidays and summer vacations.

When mom is left at a care facility, however, she never really knows for sure if she will ever see the family again.

Because it is a very sad truth that many people *are* abandoned once they move into a facility. Maybe not right away. Maybe the family will come often during the first few months. But younger people may find the place depressing, and there are always so many other things that have to be done. The visits become fewer and further between. The family comes only on holidays. Then perhaps some holidays are missed.

Nurses, aides and housekeepers who work at care facilities tell heartbreaking stories about people who have been abandoned. They liken it to best friends who are forced apart by a move. They are so miserable at first. They promise to write every day—and they do, for a while. Then they make new friends, and get busy with other things, and eventually the old dear friend is completely forgotten except, if she's lucky, for a card at Christmas. Out of sight, out of mind?

"Once the decision is made that someone will move into a care facility," Harvey Nightingale says, "the family has to develop a program for maintaining contact. The common fallacy is that the family will always be there, but the truth of the matter is that the families don't generally come.

"For the most part, many families, once they have made the placement, feel the weight of the burden removed from their shoulders, and come to visit only sporadically.

"But families should speak with the administrator about how to keep in contact with the relative, how to get involved with the residents' council, and even how to get involved with the facility as a volunteer on a regular basis."

Think of the situation of a child going off to university. What do you do? You talk on the phone all the time and visit when you can. You join the parents' group, read the school paper and newsletters, make contributions. Bake something for the annual bake sale. Attend the school plays. Put a bumper sticker on your car.

While you probably wouldn't want to put a bumper sticker on your car with the name of a care facility, the principal is the same. Your beloved family member has gone to live somewhere else, but that doesn't mean she is any less a member of the family.

"Once a person moves into a facility it becomes more difficult for the family members to remain in contact with her," says Vic Parsons, a manager for the Visiting Homemakers Association of Metropolitan Toronto. "While mother is living in her own home, it's easy to drop by after work, bring the kids over on weekends, pick her up and bring her around for dinner. It's much easier to maintain contact.

"But once she moves into a facility there are many reasons why that contact begins to diminish in many situations. Perhaps there are certain rules in terms of visiting hours, or in terms of phone calls. Perhaps you don't wish to interfere with the routine. It's pretty difficult to drop in and see mother after work, because that's the time that meals are generally being served. If she stays to see you, she might miss dinner.

"So mother starts to feel that she's less loved because she hardly ever sees the family. But it may just be because of all the barriers the facility has put up.

"But she still needs to feel she is a part of the family, and if you're not sure how to fulfill that need, then seek advice. Most of the facilities have social workers. Ask them what you can do to keep contact. Also talk with them if you've stopped visiting because you find the place so depressing. They can help you understand the situation better, and maybe see things in a different light."

Dr. Nathan Herrmann says that families should visit as often as possible, especially at the beginning. "I think they have to take the elderly relative out overnight, for afternoons, for dinner, whenever they can. A care facility is not a prison. The residents can do anything they want, you know, even go away for a weekend.

"The thing is to be involved, to show your interest. And certainly for those families who are involved and visit frequently, the relative gets better care."

Although some health professionals have disputed this, the overwhelming majority told me that this is true. And when my mother was in a nursing home, I saw it for myself.

My father visited every single day at the same time. The staff knew he would be coming, and so always had mother cleaned up and changed. The same could not be said of other residents, the great majority of whom never had any visitors.

In fact, the saddest thing about visiting there was seeing all these poor lonely people sitting out in the hallways, grabbing at us as we headed toward mother's room. They just wanted some physical contact, some human kindness.

The nurses' aides and even cleaning personnel do what they can to become the residents' new "family." Staff members often stay after their shift just to visit leisurely with people who have no visitors. They bring magazines and games from home, and often buy things like candy and cigarettes for residents who have nobody else to ask. One aide had a special relationship with one woman in the nursing home where my mother was, and she was always bringing things in for her—even dinner from McDonald's on occasion.

"In some situations," Patricia Fleming says, "where perhaps the resident is in the final stages of-Alzheimer's disease and isn't communicating and doesn't really even know where he is, visits aren't so important. But the visits are still important for the staff members, because it's essential that they know there's a family who cares about this person, and that there's someone from whom they can learn about the resident.

"Only if they know things about the resident, his previous life, his interests, what he loved to do, loved to eat, can he become a real person to the staff. Caring is so much easier if the resident is a real individual, instead of just 'a case of Alzheimer's.' By keeping in contact, the family really helps."

Dean Duncan Abraham adds: "I think one of the most important things is for family and friends to keep in touch with their loved ones once they've moved into a care facility. So many of these people feel abandoned by their families because sometimes the families get so caught up in other things. Visiting is a part of a climate we have to develop in our society—a climate of really caring for our seniors.

"This is perhaps where the church can play a role. A pastor can be a friend to people who are alone. I'm sure that if someone was in that kind of a situation and called a local clergyman, she'd find that help is available.

"Many clergy visit care facilities regularly, and take communion to those who request it, so they don't feel cut off from their church. We also spend time chatting with them if they have particular concerns. Sometimes they want to talk about practical things, like their funeral. Sometimes they have questions about death and the hereafter. I think that one of the most important parts of the pastoral ministry of any clergyman is ministering to those who are elderly and shut-in, or in care facilities, and trying to deal with their concerns and spiritual needs.

"A lot of the churches also have lay people, members of the congregation, who act as pastoral visitors and go to see people and give them a helping hand. So if someone is all alone, then the church can become family. Even if people have never gone to church, they shouldn't feel embarrassed about calling.

"In my ministry, I have always felt that if somebody comes to me for help, then my duty is to respond whether this person is a member of my congregation or not. I think you'll find that most clergy feel this way. Never be afraid to call."

Many care facility residents who do not get visitors, either because they have no family, or because the relatives they have live far away or just do not visit, depend heavily on the volunteers.

"There are so many fabulous volunteers out there," says Dr. D. William Molloy, assistant professor of medicine at McMaster University and director of the memory clinic at Henderson General Hospital in Hamilton, Ontario. "They're doing such great work. They come and give their time generously to people, and they're often not recognized for what they do.

"Many people feel that it's kind of 'sexy' to volunteer with kids, but old people are not as exciting. But it's so beautiful to go in and visit old people because they really appreciate it, and you get so much satisfaction from these visits.

"It's not hard to find volunteers to visit pediatric wings, and cancer wards. But it's difficult to convince people to visit institutions. I guess it's because people who visit care facilities see themselves there someday, and they don't want to think about it."

If there's a shortage of volunteers around the facility your relative is in, or even if there isn't, you may want to look into the possibility of hiring a companion. Even if you visit regularly, a companion can be a godsend to someone who is feeling really lonely.

Consider a companion

The best reason to hire a regular companion for your relative is that she will give her undivided attention to your relative for the time she's there. She can do whatever your relative wants or needs. One day she may read out loud, and the next she may write letters. She will also be a good listener for those times your relative just wants to talk. She may also be able to do nails, or wash and style hair. In fact, I had more than one person tell me that her mother wouldn't hardly have ever had her hair washed if it hadn't been for the companion.

If you have some very special wants, be sure to ask about them before hiring someone. You wouldn't want to have to keep changing companions, looking for someone who can do everything you require, as this would be hard on your relative. Mom might not understand why all these people keep leaving her. Companions frequently become close friends with the people they visit and are treated just like family.

Many people have companions come in for a time that covers either lunch or dinner, especially if your relative cannot eat by herself. The companion will take as long as necessary to feed her, something the aides don't always have time for.

If you can afford it, a paid companion, even for just a couple of hours a few times a week, can be the best gift you can give. It can really make a difference in the quality of your loved one's life.

Great visiting

While your loved one is still alert and getting around pretty well, visiting is easier. There are a lot of things you can do together. The key is making him feel he is still important, still a valued member of the family.

"The worst thing you can do is sit there and stare at each other," says Etta Ginsberg McEwan. "You should go out for a coffee. Maybe bring in music tapes and listen to them together. Bring in a VCR and watch a movie together. Don't feel you have to talk. In fact, you need to do more concrete things because you run out of talk.

"It's wonderful to rent or buy a video camera and make movies of things that happen at home. They don't have to be special events, just the regular happenings. This is especially important if there are little children who are growing quickly. You might also bring in photos and put them in albums together.

"Try to take your relative to as many family functions as possible to keep him involved in the lives of everyone. If he can't leave the facility because of illness, try to bring some family functions into the institution.

"Most importantly, you must tell your loved ones everything that happens at home—good, bad and even indifferent things. You have to tell them about deaths. A lot of people are afraid to tell their aging parents when someone they know has died. But you have to tell everything. You have to be able to bear with their crying if something tragic has happened in the family. This is all a part of living."

Here are some tips to make your visit great:

- Bring meaningful gifts, not things like cologne or dusting powder. Most older people have enough of those, and there generally isn't much room for storage. A few ideas—

  - Something of yourself. For example, if you bring a book, spend some time reading it out loud. Everyone in the room will enjoy this.

- A beautiful flower from your own garden, and a couple of pictures showing how great the roses were this year. Give her the opportunity of talking about the garden she used to have.

- One perfect piece of fruit, and if your relative can't feed herself, feed it to her while you're there. Don't expect the staff to have time for this.

- A favourite food. If it's something special, chances are she's not getting it at the facility. Always check with the doctor first, but if he says anything you want to bring is okay with him, then indulge your loved one. She may not have many sensuous pleasures. The best thing you can probably bring is something you've made yourself, perhaps from one of her own favourite recipes. If you can manage it, make a double batch so that others in the home can have some too. Or, if she only likes a certain kind of shortbread, or a special chocolate bar with marzipan, bring that, and do so as often as you can.

  When my father visited the nursing home where my mother was, people were always sticking dollar bills in his hand and begging him to buy them some cookies or candy. Most of these people didn't have any visitors, and so had nobody to bring them treats. Any institution's food, no matter how good, can get boring day after day. *You* enjoy treats every day; just because your relative's gotten older or sick doesn't mean she doesn't have the same desires. For just a couple of dollars each time you visit, you can bring something that will be really appreciated.

- A lunch fresh from your relative's favourite fast-food place, especially if the facility always serves something she hates on Thursdays. Seniors love fast food just as much as anybody else.

- Craft supplies. If your relative was always active and is still able to do a lot of things, the activities at the facility may not be satisfying for her. These activities are generally pretty simple, so that everyone can participate. But if your mother was an expert knitter, or was involved in some other more intricate craft, she may really be missing it. Bring her some pattern books to look at, and if she expresses interest, pick up some yarn and supplies. Even if your mother or aunt wasn't a great needleworker, you might be able to get her interested in such activity now. Life can get pretty boring with nothing to do but watch TV. Bring her some beautiful yarn and a crochet hook big enough to be easily held. Show her just one simple stitch.

This is also one of the best ways to give your relative some independence. She could knit or crochet up a bunch of afghans, socks or sweaters and then give them to family members and friends for Christmas or birthdays. Nobody could refuse such a beautiful and loving gift. All you have to do is keep her supplied with yarn and patterns. This sure beats her having to ask someone to *buy* gifts for her to give to people.

- Drawings from the little ones in the family. (Not all gifts have to cost money.) Some residents' walls are covered with them.

- Old magazines or clippings you think she'll be interested in. Read them to her.

- Subscriptions to a couple of her favourite magazines. Other people may bring in old issues, but it's really special to have your own copy, to be the first one to see a nice new magazine that nobody's ripped anything out of yet.

- Embossed writing paper. If writing is a problem for her, let her dictate letters to you. Try to do this as often as you can. It will help her keep in touch with friends she's left behind— and when she sends letters, she will get letters. It's sad for mail call to come and go day after day with never anything for you.

- Yourself and your time, probably the best gift you can give. Visit as often as you can. Tell jokes. Tell family gossip. Play "remember when."

- Read the Bible together and talk about it, or pray together. If your loved one was very religious all her life, just because she can't get out to church now doesn't mean she is any less religious. She may have a deep need for some spiritual food, and will really appreciate your supplying it.

- Bring people along with you when you visit, especially old family friends. Just don't bring too many people at one time, especially if your loved one is not feeling well. Keep visits short and sweet.

- Try to organize the timing of visits of the family members so that weeks don't go by with nobody coming, and then everybody coming all at once. If fifteen people visit on Mother's Day, it may be too overwhelming for mom and just tire her out. She would probably much prefer fifteen separate visits.

- Make visits short and often. Ten fifteen-minute visits are better than one two-hour visit.

- Tell her when you'll next be coming to create anticipation. She'll be all dressed up and ready. If life is dull, you can't imagine how much people look forward to visitors.

- Focus on special days, like birthdays and anniversaries. Be sure to do something special on these days. Most care facilities have large rooms where you can throw a party. Invite the whole family. Invite the other residents and the staff. Really make it a day to remember. Mom will talk about it all year long.

- Ask the head nurse if you can bring your pet for a visit. If you have a friendly well-behaved pet, this is one of the best things you can do for everyone in the facility. You'll see people light up when they touch something soft, warm and furry again.

- Be a good listener, no matter how many times dad tells the same old stories. Many people cannot remember what they had for breakfast, but can vividly recall the past.

- Let him complain about his situation. Talking about problems will help. If you feel something should be done about the complaints, tell him you'll look into them. Never promise that you'll take care of everything, because you may not be able to.

- Let him express his feelings, even if they're always sad. He may have had to give up a lot when he moved into the facility, and it may take a while to get over this. It's a mistake to make light of his feelings and tell him he'll just "get over it." Never talk to him like to a child. His feelings are just as legitimate as they ever were. *He* didn't change when he changed his address.

- If mom doesn't always look her best because the staff is too busy to spend extra time with her, you can help with some of these things. Bring fresh clothes and help her change. You can wash and set her hair, do her nails. You can even do more important things, such as brushing her teeth and helping her to the bathroom. She may be in diapers all the rest of the time, but if she can go to the bathroom herself, allow her this dignity when you're there. She'll feel a hundred times better about herself.

- Try to have a positive attitude. Put yourself in the resident's place and ask yourself what you would like and how you would like to be treated. Remember that even though your relative may be ill, his mind may be just fine, in fact, maybe better than yours!

- The other residents now make up part of your relative's community. So treat them with kindness and respect. Make an effort to get to know them, learn their names. Many of them are lonely, many have no visitors, and many have no family at all. Don't be discouraged if people don't warm to you immediately. It may take time, but persevere. People often become quite self-absorbed when they have nothing to do but think about their problems and aches and pains all day. So don't just commiserate with everybody when you visit—try to get their minds on something else.

- Bring the little ones when you visit. Many people don't, because they fear that the noise will upset the residents, or that the children will be disturbed at the sight of so many sick people. But in fact, this is a way for children to learn to deal with aging and illness. Besides, elderly residents love to see children.

- Be sure your loved one stays in touch with old friends, churches and the community. Offer to pick up friends and take them home if it will help them visit more often. Anything you can do to keep your relative in touch will diminish the sense of isolation he may feel.

- Instead of just idle chatter, try to enhance mom's self-esteem by making her feel wanted and needed. Take samples of wallpaper and ask for her help in choosing the one for the kitchen. Let her help plan a party. Ask dad for advice on insurance or fishing.

- Don't try to hide family problems and other bad news. Ask for help and advice when you can. Older people have a lot to contribute, and their helping you cope with a crisis increases their self-esteem.

- If your relative doesn't always recognize friends and family members, introduce yourself and others each time you visit.

- People in comas are often aware of visitors. Ask the doctor for advice on how to communicate with them.

To sum up . . .

- Many people fear abandonment once they've moved into a care facility.

- Keeping in touch can be hard sometimes. In some cases, you have too much to do already, and in others the facility puts up barriers to easy visiting and communication.

- Nothing is sadder than someone who waits and waits for a call or a visit, but nothing comes.

- The suggestions above come from a lot of caring people. With a little creativity, you can think of twice as many.

- The key is keeping your loved one a part of the family, no matter how old or sick she or he may be getting. Everyone has a right to the same respect and consideration they did before changing addresses.

CHAPTER ELEVEN

KEEPING AN EYE ON THE FOOD

I f you've ever been a patient in a hospital, you know how bored you can get. You look forward to mealtimes in a way you might never do at home, simply because a meal may be the high point of the day. The same applies to those in a care facility, and maybe even more so. Mealtime may be the residents' main source of stimulation and pleasure. And for those who can go to the dining room, it's also a social event. A resident may spend most of the day alone, but at mealtimes he can get together with others and talk.

For those who are stuck in their rooms, this is a time for direct one-on-one care and personal contact from the person who feeds them.

So if you want to make sure that your loved one is being well taken care of in a facility, looking at the food is a good place to start. Although it wouldn't be fair to say that the best places have the best food, you can get a good indication of how much love and care is put into taking care of the residents by looking at the quality of the food and how it's prepared and served.

As a registered professional dietitian, Patricia Crane is a consultant to nursing homes and in nutrition for the elderly. I asked her for some advice in this area.

"There are definite rules in regard to nursing homes following Canada's Food Guide and making sure that the menus are set up without repetition," she says. "It is recommended that nursing homes have consulting dietitians, but a lot of them try to avoid it because they don't want the expense. Inspectors check the menus and inspect the premises, but you don't really know what happens between inspections on a day-to-day basis. It's hoped they're following the rules and regulations, but they may not always.

"If you have a relative in a nursing home, I think being around at mealtime is important. Nutritious menus with lots of variety are a part of nursing-home regulations, but these menus may not always be followed and the food not always be prepared in a manner acceptable to the residents. If you don't like what you see, my biggest word of advice is, be vocal and make the dietary and nursing staff aware of the dietary needs of your relative—his likes and dislikes.

"Be sure to tell them what alternative the resident might like if he doesn't want what is on the menu. Be sure they know if he has any allergies, or if there is anything about certain foods that the dietary people need to know. They generally just prepare one basic meal and everybody gets basically the same thing if they are not on a special diet.

"But there is always supposed to be an alternative available. For instance, if they prepare chicken today, and your mother doesn't like chicken or is allergic to chicken, then she should be able to tell them that, and something else should be provided. But the only way that the alternative would get to the resident is if there's communication."

The food-service supervisor or dietary personnel should be available to speak with the residents and the families. If they are not, and you have to speak to a nurse or aide, then one of the biggest problems is seeing that your comments reach the right person so that changes can be made.

Everybody wants to eat what they like, and they also want to have a choice. Most nursing homes have residents' councils, and the meetings provide an opportunity for all residents to have input into the meals. Usually that's the time when the residents get to choose their menus or the things they like. It's also a chance for them to express dissatisfactions.

For example, Ms. Crane told me about one nursing home where they were always trying to do all kinds of fancy things with potatoes, but the residents were finding the results hard or dry. So a request was made through the residents' council for just plain mashed potatoes. Residents didn't want variety in the way the potatoes were prepared; they just wanted plain well-mashed potatoes that were good and easy to eat.

You'll find that most care facilities are responsive to this kind of request. But they can't do anything unless the residents make their needs known. Harvey Nightingale told me about one nursing home where every Thursday one of the dinner choices was "wieners and beans." The government inspector said that wasn't an appropriate option, so they stopped serving it. Well, the residents rebelled! They wanted their wieners and beans, and didn't care what the government said. Communication is vital.

If you visit the facility for several days at dinnertime and see every meal, and each one is worse than the other, what should you do?

Ms. Crane recommends that you go to the administrator of the home, or if he's not there, the person in authority at that time. Ask if you may speak to the food-service supervisor or the dietitian about the meals.

"You could give your message to the administrator," she says, "but I think it's better to go directly to the person who's responsible for preparing the meals. Because sometimes the messages don't always get through from the administrator, or they're watered down before they reach the person responsible."

Sometimes problems result because there is a lot of turnover in the kitchen staff. If there are always new people, they don't get to know the residents and what they like.

And in the large facilities there's sometimes very little contact between the residents and the staff. Let's say it's a large home with the kitchen in the basement, and the meals go up to the dining floor on trays on a lift. It's the nurse's aides who make sure that the residents get the right trays, and that they get fed.

In these large facilities, the food-service supervisor may not have any direct contact with the residents at all. So you may find that a smaller facility offers better food because there's closer contact, and the residents know exactly what's going on in the kitchen. The bigger the facility, the less opportunity there may be for communication and individuality in the meals.

But even in a large facility, if the staff is good at communicating and the supervisor is responsible and caring, you can still get results. The fact that a facility is large doesn't mean lack of good care there—but it can mean a greater chance of poor communication; interaction between dietary staff and residents is more difficult.

The main contact is the food-service supervisor, though, and if she doesn't come around regularly and the nurses aren't interested or don't bother communicating requests and complaints, then chances are the residents aren't getting exactly what they want.

What should you do if your loved one is always complaining about the food? The best advice I got from everyone is to be sure to visit at meal-time—several, not just once or twice. Most places will be glad to serve you a meal so that you can eat with your relative, although there's usually a charge.

It's especially nice to join your loved one for the main meal on special days, such as Thanksgiving, Christmas and birthdays, if you can't bring him home to eat with the family. But don't judge the everyday food by what they serve then. If you come several times over a two- or three-week period, you'll see better what the food is actually like.

When you visit at meal-time to check out your relative's complaints, have a good look around. Don't just stay in his room. See that all the residents are actually eating. Or if they can't eat themselves, that they are being fed the meals, and that they are being fed when the food is still hot and palatable. There should be enough staff to start feeding the residents the minute the trays are delivered. If all the trays have to be delivered down four long hallways before staff members get back to start feeding the people who got the trays first, perhaps thirty minutes later, you might want to say something about this to the supervisor.

It's also important that the residents have enough time to eat. Sometimes you'll see the staff, as soon as they've finished moving up the hall passing out meals to those who can feed themselves, they go back down the hall and start collecting the trays from the first ones served. This is probably not enough time for people to finish. The trays should be left as long as there's a chance people will eat more.

It's another story for those who cannot feed themselves. If the facility is short-staffed, you may notice each resident getting only a few mouthfuls before the person feeding him has to move on to the next room.

If you see this happening to other residents and suspect it is happening to your relative—a good sign can also be a dramatic weight loss—you must say something.

If you don't want to say anything, you can do what my father did—he simply visited every single day at dinnertime and fed my mother himself. Sometimes it took an hour, because one of the symptoms of her disease was that she would take a mouthful of food, and just chew and chew until someone told her ten times to swallow it. He doubts that anyone on the staff would have had this much time and patience to give her every evening, and I think he was right. I fed my mother a few times, and believe me, it was exhausting.

If you cannot personally always be there to feed your loved one every meal, pull together the resources of the family. Make up a schedule. If you have enough willing relatives and friends, each of you may only get feeding duty once every three or four weeks.

Or if you have the money, you can always hire a companion to come in at mealtimes. Several people found that having a companion from just before lunch until just after dinner was the best time. Then they were assured the resident got two full meals.

Even if there is enough staff to make sure that meals are served hot and that everyone has enough time to eat, there is the food itself to consider. If your relative is always complaining, be sure to order several meals for yourself and give the food an honest try—you can't always tell by just looking.

The only things my mother seemed to really enjoy from the trays were the milk and the puddings, on the rare occasions that they had pudding. So my father started bringing a pudding cup every single day when he visited, so that she always had something she liked.

If the food is simply bland, you can help by bringing in a few spices or condiments from home if it's all right with your relative's doctor. Since the facility is cooking for a lot of people, you have to expect that the food wouldn't be salted or spiced much.

But if the meat is gray and mostly fat, the potatoes undercooked and dry, and the fruit bruised or mouldy, you have legitimate grounds for complaint. And be sure to do so. Not only for the sake of your loved one, but also for the sake of all the other residents who may not have anyone there to speak up for them.

People in facilities really look forward to meals, sometimes lining up an hour before time. And it's only fair that their meals are good. The enjoyment of a meal may be one of the few pleasures they have left.

On top of that, it breaks your heart to see these old and frail people so thin. They sometimes look as if they would break if you sneezed in their direction. People should be encouraged to eat, if for no other reason than to keep up their body weight and their strength. And of course the best way to do that is to have really good food available to them.

Most facilities in Canada have tuck-shops where residents can buy books and magazines, treats like chocolate and snacks, and personal-care items like toothbrushes. If someone cannot get to the shop, another resident or a staff member will usually be happy to pick something up for him. Even if a resident's entire pension goes to paying the nursing home, he is still given a "comfort allowance." This gives him a little personal money to spend as he pleases.

You might, as my father was, be tempted to bring in treats for other residents. Just be sure to check with the nurse or doctor first. You wouldn't want to give cookies to someone with diabetes, for instance. If you can afford it, you might want to bring in enough for everybody on your relative's wing once in a while—perhaps a big cake, or several bags of cookies. The nurses will see that all of those who can have this kind of treat get some.

The woman who shared the room with my mother was without family and all alone in the world. She loved popcorn, and it was her greatest enjoyment in life. So every Friday my father brought her one of those huge bags of popcorn. He called it payment for her keeping an eye on mother, and so the woman never felt it was charity. Even after my mother died, he used to visit her at least once a month and bring her some popcorn, because he knew nobody else would.

Most homes do have treats for the residents, and what they have and when depends on budget constraints and how willing the staff is to make the extra effort. Most places will have perhaps cookies and juice in the afternoon. But check—does each person get only one small glass of juice and one cookie? What if they want more?

If you've noticed your relative appears to have had a serious weight loss, by all means speak to the doctor. However, if your mother's greatest joy in life was cooking and baking, and eating her creations, she might have been overweight when she came into the home. This would certainly explain some weight loss.

But if she's always complaining about being hungry, and always begging you to bring in things, I'd definitely have a talk with the doctor.

Ms. Crane told me that the kitchen staff at most of the homes she consults for are thrilled when somebody really loves the food and asks for seconds or thirds. They love to give extra food to the people who really enjoy and want it. I think it should be that way everywhere.

But if you do notice that your relative is losing a lot of weight and she wasn't particularly overweight to begin with, you must ask the doctor about it. In some cases it will be because of the food; in other cases it may be a sign of whatever disease she has. Some diseases cause wasting away, and some cause people to lose their sense of taste and smell, so they don't desire food. Some medical problems and treatments also cause nausea, so people don't want to eat. There is an explanation.

If the weight loss is caused by bad food, not enough time to eat, or not enough food, you can and must speak out. Be very vocal. You'll not only be helping your loved one, but everyone else who will ever have to be a resident of that facility.

If the weight loss is caused by a disease or treatment, you should suggest to the doctor that supplemental feeding be done before it gets too bad. My mother wasted away to almost nothing before my father spoke to someone about it, because he thought that was just the way it had to be with cancer patients. But we asked to attend one of the care meetings they had about the patients, and when we did, we asked if something could be done. They started supplemental feeding that very day.

Dr. Alastair Cunningham, program director for the Ontario Cancer Institute, wonders why they didn't do this for my mother sooner. "The usual practice," he states, "is to do everything possible to get food into patients, even if they're clearly dying, and even if it means intravenous feeding. That should normally be done.

"If family members see their loved one wasting away to nothing, they should certainly request that supplemental feeding be started. There may in some cases be contra-indications, medical reasons why it shouldn't be done, but they can request strongly. If the family makes their wants known, and the patient isn't obviously opposed, there's no question that it should be done—even if it means hospitalization and feeding intravenously."

All residents should be weighed regularly once a month, and if they seem to be losing weight rapidly, it should be every week. This weight loss should be pointed out to a doctor, and he should prescribe supplemental feeding before things get bad. But if this system breaks down, as it did in my mother's case, you must speak up.

The recreational directors at most facilities do what they can, within budgetary restrictions of course, to arrange special-treat nights for residents. Most places have pizza nights at least once a month, as residents, like everybody else, love pizza. I've also been told of a couple of places that occasionally have special nights where everyone gets really dressed up, and they not only have a special dinner, but wine too.

There are a lot of other special nights that can be arranged without much cost. Pub nights are ever popular, as are ethnic nights. German night can have not only German food, but also oom-pah-pah music and decorations.

Some homes have buffets on a regular basis, so that residents really get to choose what they want and how much they want. The people who cannot walk through the buffet on their own are helped to select what they want by staff and other residents first, and then the people who can help themselves eat.

If there's a patio, in good weather lunch or an afternoon treat can be served there like a picnic.

When I worked for a while as an activities director in a hospital psychiatric ward, I used to bring in my ice-cream maker every Thursday and we'd all make ice cream together in the afternoon—a different flavour each week, chosen by popular vote. I honestly think that this was the high point of the week for a lot of people—some would be sitting in the room hours before time.

I asked Patricia Crane if someone ever just goes out to a popular burger place to bring in dinner on occasion. If I were in a facility, I know this is one thing I would miss the most. She said that the idea has been tried by some homes, but it didn't work out as well as hoped. Several staff members would have to leave the facility at the same time to pick up the food, which would have caused a problem in an emergency, and by the time they returned and passed everything out, the food was usually cold and soggy. Some people didn't mind—it was still a treat.

Most facilities make up special treats such as cakes for birthdays, especially if it's a milestone birthday. Larger facilities may have one celebration each month for all the people who had birthdays that month, with one big cake for everybody.

Ms. Crane also told me about a very special treat the staff at one facility gives to a certain man who has no family. On his birthday they take him out to dinner wherever he wants. The staff chips in and he gets a big meal—whatever he wants, with no regard to cost. They do this because he's diabetic, so he can't have a cake. He has a ball on this day. He gets to eat exactly what he wants, but it's more than that. It's an outing, and this means a lot to him because he so seldom gets out and sees anyone.

If the staff seems a little less than creative in its approach to special-treat days, it certainly wouldn't hurt to make some recommendations to them. Or even better, if you have a little time you can plan one yourself. It really takes very little to make so many people happy.

My uncle and aunt are in a nursing home, although not the same one my mother was in. Every Christmas my cousin Doris, their niece, dresses her boss up in a Santa suit and brings him by the home. He's a portly fellow, and he makes a big deal of his role. He laughs a loud jolly laugh that can be heard throughout the building, and everyone runs up to see him. He hands out candy canes to everyone, staff and residents alike.

This is a very simple thing to arrange. It costs very little and takes only a couple of hours. But people talked about Santa for months afterward. For many of them, it was the only personal contact they had with anyone at Christmas, or even the whole year.

With only a little creativity your friends and family can come up with some great ideas too. One woman told me about how she brought in a piper to serenade her mother, a Scot, on her birthday. Everyone enjoyed it, because it was something really different.

It may be best to plan things for times other than Christmas, as many organizations and schools take care of arranging special treats in facilities at Christmas. Birthdays are an obvious choice for a good time, but it's also nice to do something for no reason at all.

Just check with the head nurse to make sure that something else isn't planned for the same day. Then bring in the whole family, especially the little ones, and throw a party.

To sum up...

- The quality of the food and how it's prepared and served is a good indication of the level of love and care for the residents in a facility.

- If the food is really awful, you must say something—not only for your loved one, but also for the sake of all those who may not have anyone to speak up for them.

- If there are serious problems, such as the staff not taking enough time to feed residents properly, or not allowing them enough time to eat on their own, you must say something.

- If your requests fall on deaf ears, see Chapter 14, Getting action on your complaints. Never be afraid to fight for better food, as this may be the only pleasure many residents have.

- Take just a little time to plan and throw a special event for all the residents who share life with your loved one. Bring something wonderful in the way of food and entertainment—and don't forget to invite the staff.

CHAPTER TWELVE

MEDICAL AND DENTAL CONCERNS

Just because your loved one has gone into a care facility does not mean that she will be taken care of in every aspect. Although you may want her to have the best possible care, which you are no longer able to provide, this is seldom possible in an institutional setting, no matter how pleasant or expensive the place may be.

Staff shortages, some of them severe, cause most of the problems. Because no matter how dedicated the staff is, there just aren't enough hands to do all the work. If you've cared for your relative, you know how much care one person requires. Multiply that by a hundred or five hundred, however many there are in the facility.

So although you may breathe a little easier because the burden of giving care is not squarely on your shoulders anymore, your job is not finished. You still have to keep an eye on things to make sure that your relative's basic and most important needs are met. And if the staff can't seem to get to everything, you may have to pitch in yourself, or hire a paid companion to help out.

Your most important job is keeping tabs on medical and dental needs. Because no matter how good the food is, or how pretty the flower garden is, those things are not the most important. Health is. Someone who does not have his basic health needs met won't give a hoot about the food or the flowers.

Dr. Duncan Robertson believes that a family physician with an interest in care of the elderly is probably the most important asset for the long-term care of a frail older person. Each person needs a physician who is willing to visit him in the care facility, and not just to handle emergencies. I would ask the head nurse if it's possible for your relative to keep seeing the same doctor he has known for years, if the doctor will visit. Some places will not allow this, so always ask first, before you approach the doctor.

If this is okay with the facility, ask your relative's doctor if he would be willing to make a routine trip to the facility at least four times a year to see him, and also if he would be available to go there in case of an emergency. Many people feel that this is the most ideal situation, because he has known your relative and his problems for years, and would be the best person to take care of him.

Many doctors are happy to continue your loved one's care and, in fact, if the facility is nearby, he may already have several patients there that he visits. Many doctors are unwilling to do this, however, and will turn over the care of a patient to the staff doctor as soon as someone enters a facility.

In some long-term-care facilities there is a staff doctor or physician who makes regular visits and who has under his or her care a large number of the residents of that facility. And some places will insist you use this physician. This may be more convenient to some families and patients, but it may mean changing care from a physician who the older person has known and trusted for years.

It is important for a new doctor taking over the medical care of a resident, to have access to information about the resident's previous health, operations and drug treatments. This information should be obtained from the resident's previous physician, and from previous hospital or health-care facility's records.

If you're encouraged to have a private physician take care of mom, but the doctor she's had for years is unwilling, you'll have to find someone else. Family members who are looking for a new physician should ask questions about his training in geriatrics, and of course his willingness to make visits to the facility.

The physician should be willing to make regular visits. The kinds of medical care required by the frail elderly are obviously determined by each person's health problems, but Dr. Duncan Robertson recommends quarterly routine visits. At these times the medical care and drug therapy can be reviewed.

It's particularly important to keep an eye on the medications residents are taking. Many older people take different kinds of pills for all different kinds of problems, and these have to be monitored.

Often, once a person enters a facility, some of his medication can be cut back or stopped. This is because of the consistent, regular care he gets in the facility.

Regular nourishing meals and regular on-time administration of medications can improve some conditions. People living alone may not always eat properly and may often forget to take their pills. So once they're being taken care of, things can improve dramatically.

Some new residents may be given a sedative to help them cope with the anxiety caused by moving out of their own homes and into a facility. But after a month or so, they are usually able to stop this medication because they have adjusted. Nothing is sadder than to go into a care facility where the residents are all slumped over and looking like zombies because of too much sedation. In most cases, this is absolutely unnecessary.

If you want to know what medications your loved one is being given, just ask the head nurse. If you don't understand the fancy names, ask her to explain what each drug is for. If you think your relative is getting too much medication, or an inappropriate one, by all means ask the doctor about it.

Likewise, if you think your relative has other problems that aren't being treated, be sure to ask about that, too. For example, depression is common among older people, but many doctors don't want to give drugs for this. If you think anti-depressants might help bring about a little better quality of life, ask the doctor. (See Chapter 13, Depression among people in care situations.)

Don't forget that residents of care facilities have the right to refuse any medications. But in order to do this, they need to know what they are taking. If your mother complains that she has absolutely no energy since she entered the facility, she may be depressed—or, the staff may be giving her sedatives without her knowing. Once it's known that it's a drug causing the problem, this drug can be refused.

Another consideration is pain. "There are a number of conditions that cause long-standing pain in older people," says Dr. Robertson, "and these chronically painful conditions can indeed lead to both distress and despondency, as well as limitation in function. The problem with medications used for pain is that, while they're effective, they also have adverse effects—and the older person is much more liable to encounter adverse effects from medications. They may be as simple as constipation, or they may be as serious as ulcers, which can be fatal.

"So when a person has a life expectancy of three to five years, and the use of medications may compromise their self-care abilities and their enjoyment of life, then the physician, the patient and the care givers together have to make some difficult judgements as to the appropriate use of medication. It may be impossible to render a patient totally free of pain without impairing his level of consciousness, and thus impairing his enjoyment of life."

Dr. Jack Lee and Dr. Mary Kudrac point out that an important dental problem facing seniors, especially those in nursing homes, is the loss of dentures. And the reason is that they are not labelled. Every denture when it's made should have the patient's name on it, and if this isn't done at the time of manufacture, the name can be put on later. When you are living alone losing dentures isn't a problem, but in an institution with a hundred other denture wearers, it is. The elderly, who are often a bit forgetful, end up leaving them on the food trays or losing them in the bed linen. And when the dentures turn up somewhere else, there is no way of reuniting them with their owner if no name is on them.

There's another common way dentures get lost. When you are ill and an ambulance takes you to a hospital, the first thing they do is remove your dentures. One of the saddest things many doctors told me is coming across people who move into the institution with dentures only to have them lost later, and then not being able to have those dentures replaced.

"Many times," says Dr. Lee, "I have come to see a woman who doesn't have her dentures and I ask her what happened, and then the tears start. She tells me that she got ill, was taken to the hospital, and the dentures were lost. And she has no way of getting them replaced. It takes just a few minutes to put the name on the dentures, and it can prevent tragedy later on. If the name is there, even if the dentures are lost at the hospital, they can be reunited later with the owner back at the nursing home."

Lack of dental care is a problem in a care facility, and the oral health of seniors does suffer. Dr. Lee explained that nursing-home administration is very much aware of this problem and appreciates any support in improving this situation. The reason seniors' teeth and dentures are neglected in nursing homes is staff shortage. They're very busy places, what with bathing and feeding and all, so things that may be considered a little less important often have to take a back seat because there just isn't time to do everything.

And for the most part staff members are not knowledgeable enough about proper mouth care or its importance, so as a result they're not motivated. They also find mouth care a very unpleasant duty.

If you see that your loved one's oral hygiene is being neglected at a care facility, what should you do?

First, you should immediately raise your concerns with the care givers. Tell them how important your relative's dental care is.

The individuals who are more or less physically able can brush their teeth or remove and clean their dentures themselves. But even then, the staff should remind them to do so.

Many of the people in institutions are cognitively impaired, and that's why they are there. They often just get confused and forget that it's been two or three days since they brushed their teeth or taken out their dentures. These people especially need daily reminders. For those individuals who are physically compromised and not able to take care of their own mouths, the family must talk with the administrators and staff, and make sure someone is assigned routinely to do this task. Otherwise the lack of care will lead to degeneration, pain and infection.

Family members can also lobby for regular visits from their local public-health unit. While some health units in Canada do this on a regular basis, there aren't enough. If outside political pressure is put on the local public-health to make regular visits, it would go a long way to improving the situation for all the seniors in facilities.

Public-health officers could provide preventive clinical services, such as cleaning teeth and removing tartar. They could also educate, both the residents capable of doing their own hygiene, and the staff.

It's important that family members make sure their loved one has her own toothbrush, her own denture cup, and her name on her dentures. Make sure that her name is written with indelible ink on the denture cup and the toothbrush, and while you're at it, see that her name is put on eyeglasses or any other personal item. Because in a nursing-home situation things get lost.

And as one resident said, since he's physically unable to leave the facility to buy himself a new toothbrush, the one he has is an extremely important thing.

Each week or so, when you visit, you should look at your relative's mouth. It's as simple as checking to see if the teeth are clean or if there is a build-up of calculus or tartar, or if the gums look kind of dirty.

If dad wears dentures, check the inside of his mouth. If there is debris there, the dentures probably are not being cleaned regularly. And if that's the case, you should go directly to the staff or the administrator, and find out why. If they're not clean it means someone is not doing her job—either not ensuring that the resident is taking daily care of his mouth, or not giving the necessary assistance.

Family members should check for proper mouth care just as carefully as they would make sure a resident is getting his proper medication, or not developing bedsores. If you find that grandma seems to be suffering from her medication or that bedsores are developing and not being taken care of, you should go to the staff immediately and demand that proper care be given—and the same thing applies to mouth care. A dirty mouth, or bleeding gums, or grimy dentures, or even a missing toothbrush, all should be treated like any other important health issue.

Just because someone is aging does not mean he has to lose more teeth. No matter what his age, a person doesn't lose teeth unless his teeth and gums are not being properly taken care of. But it becomes more difficult for those who go into institutions when they are physically or cognitively impaired, and unable to do the job themselves. This is where family members have to exert pressure on the guardians—the institution staff.

If you notice that granddad is not wearing his dentures, ask why. First of all ask where they are, or if they have been lost. Or is he reluctant to wear them because they're painful? Sometimes a sore in the mouth caused by a denture rubbing against the gum is extremely painful, but it's a simple problem that can be fixed by a dentist in minutes. So find out why these dentures are not being worn.

Good dental health means freedom from pain. You can't get enjoyment out of life unless you are free of pain. Good dental health also means the ability to chew. In the elderly, eating is often one of the last remaining pleasures. Old age is an age of loss, and many seniors are physically unable to do a lot of things they once enjoyed, but eating seems to be the one thing that is left. Lack of good dental health takes that enjoyment away, and they are relegated to a life of eating mush.

Lastly, looking and smelling good is important to everybody regardless of age. "One of the saddest stories I ever came across," Dr. Kudrac says, "is when an elderly resident opened up to me and confessed that the reason he refused invitations to his daughter-in-law's home for family dinners was that he was embarrassed by his lack of teeth and his poor dental health. He didn't want to make his grandchildren and the rest of the family uncomfortable around the dinner table. So lack of dental health in this case denied him a very important interaction with his family."

To sum up. . .

- Medical and dental care is just as important in a care facility as it is anywhere else.

- Even if someone is old and near the end of his life, he is still entitled to good medical and dental care to make his remaining time as enjoyable as possible.

- If you think your relative isn't being properly seen to, talk to the staff and the administrator. The solution is usually simple.

CHAPTER THIRTEEN
DEPRESSION AMONG PEOPLE IN CARE SITUATIONS

Depression among the elderly, both men and women, is very common. In fact elderly men have the highest rate of "successful" suicide of any age and sex group. Depression is scientifically categorized into major—called clinical depression—and minor forms.

About two to five per cent of people over sixty-five suffer from clinical depression, and an additional ten per cent may have mild depression. Sunnybrook Health Science Centre psychiatrist Dr. Ivan L. Silver believes that about five to ten per cent of people in long-term-care facilities may suffer from clinical depression at any point in time.

Doctors generally agree that clinical depression requires treatment, and in fact the success of anti-depressant drugs has led to a change in the understanding of depressive illness and how the brain works. However, there is a fair amount of controversy concerning the treatment of or the approach to the patient with minor depression. It's not clear if minor depression responds to medication.

Families of patients who are depressed often try to help them by encouraging them, reassuring them, even gently pushing them to get up and do things. When these manoeuvres don't work, professional help should be called in.

Sometimes the family will have to work hard to get their elderly relative to see a counsellor or psychiatrist. In fact, the depressed person may have given up all hope of getting better or feeling better and will call the family's efforts pointless.

"Whenever somebody loses interest in his usual activities, does not seem to be able to enjoy things he used to and seems rather slowed down in activity," says Dr. M. Oluwafemi Agbayewa, "you must talk about depression. If in addition to this or instead of this the person also has difficulty sleeping, especially if he wakes up earlier in the morning than usual and has difficulty getting back to sleep, or loses his appetite, then depression should be considered.

"Occasionally you will find individuals who are depressed who tend to sleep all the time, much more than they need, and eat more than usual and sometimes put on weight. The important thing about the sleep and appetite is that there is a change in the usual patterns. It doesn't matter which direction the change is in.

"Other symptoms include social isolation, not wanting to or not being interested in relating to friends, cutting down social engagements and staying alone all the time. These can also be related to other illnesses, especially limiting conditions. So that's why it's important to have a professional assessment."

Dr. Silver lists the following warning signs of someone possibly developing a depression, one that should be looked at:

- A recent change of overall mood, including complaints of feeling depressed, anxious or nervous

- Change in appetite, including recent weight loss or gain

- Decreased energy, decreased ambition

- Decreased concentration

- Increasingly morbid view of himself and the world

- Increased expression of guilt

- Increased preoccupation with health and worrying about becoming ill

- Increased preoccupation with his body

- More than usual ramblings about trivial matters

- A sense of hopelessness and helplessness

- Mentions of suicide

"Whenever a person complains of helplessness or hopelessness," adds Dr. Agbayewa, "these should be taken seriously, because they often precede suicidal behaviour. Of course any verbalization of the intent to kill oneself to rejoin a lost loved one, or a preoccupation with the hereafter, then immediate assistance should be sought."

Dr. Yoel Isenberg thinks depression is something that should be looked at on a variety of levels. For one, you must make sure that it is depression and not another condition such as agitation, anxiety, confusion or a normal reaction to various stresses such as the death of a loved one.

"It's also important that there aren't underlying medical conditions that can cause depression," he says. "There are many conditions, including a variety of viral illnesses, such as infectious mononucleosis and hepatitis, and a variety of other metabolic and hormonal abnormalities, that may be easily treatable. And of course there are more tragic conditions, such as cancer of the pancreas and brain tumors, that can cause depression. It's important to establish a diagnosis first, because the ideal treatment would be to treat the underlying condition that is causing depression.

"A person who is first diagnosed as being depressed in late life may very well have an underlying neurologic problem. That problem may be a stroke, which very commonly causes depression. Whether or not the person recovers from the stroke, the depression may respond to anti-depressant medication. Depression may also be due to a brain tumor, and the brain tumor is not treatable. In any case it's always appropriate to look for an underlying diagnosis and then consider whether or not the depression itself can be treated."

Once the diagnosis and underlying conditions are established, the doctor can decide whether to treat the depression itself, and how. It's important also to address the human and emotional context in which the depression arises. For example, a man who is retired after working his entire adult life and who never had hobbies, may require some guidance or counselling in order to handle the abundance of leisure time he suddenly has. He may be moping around simply because of boredom, nothing to do or nothing to interest him.

A person who is grieving may also seem depressed, so it's important to understand the stages of mourning for a lost loved one to be able to differentiate what is considered normal and pathological bereavement. And remember, someone's moving out of his home and into a care facility may also cause grieving, because a spouse may be left behind. Many people go into mourning in situations like this, even if the spouse has not died. If you think this may be the problem, you should ask that a counsellor or social worker come in for a talk. Medication is not called for in all cases of depression. Many times, counselling itself will make all the difference in the quality of someone's life.

Clinical depression isn't caused just by being in a nursing home when you don't want to be there, and feeling that your life is over, and that this home is so depressing, and you know this is all you have for the rest of your life. That's just a depressing *situation*. And it's important to bear in mind that people who are in nursing homes are there because they have to be.

Twenty years ago it was very common to find people in their sixties in nursing homes. Nowadays we find people in their sixties and seventies coming to visit their parents in nursing homes. The people who reside in these homes now are not only much older than before, but much sicker.

"It's true that many doctors do not recognize depression in the elderly," Dr. Isenberg thinks. "Depression is a common condition that rarely comes to the attention of psychiatrists. Most emotional conditions are brought to the attention of the family physician, if anyone.

However, there are detailed surveys that indicate that many elderly people never discuss their emotions with any health-care personnel. They are more reluctant to express their feelings or to say something like, 'Hey doc, I really feel down in the dumps.'

"That may be because people who are now in their eighties grew up in a time when feelings were not as freely expressed as they are today. It may be that these people do not consider themselves depressed, but their depression may be manifested by a variety of somatic symptoms such as abdominal pain, constipation, headache, and so on. They may not experience a feeling of sadness and may resist the notion that their persistent headache—assuming that various neurologic causes of headache have been considered and eliminated—is in fact a manifestation of depression not perceived as such by the patient. It's also true that there are many family physicians who are not sensitive to the prevalence and treatability of depression."

Dr. Isenberg tells the story of an eighty-year-old woman who goes to her physician complaining of pain in one knee. This pain has persisted and is clearly impairing her ability to walk and be independent. After examining her and finding nothing striking on physical examination, the physician says, "Well Mrs. X, what do you want? You've been walking on that knee for eighty years and there's a lot of wear and tear. You wouldn't expect your car to last eighty years, and it's made of steel. That's just the way it is."

Mrs. X responds, "But my other knee is also eighty years old and it doesn't hurt."

The message is that age in and of itself does not inevitably cause disease. It is important to always keep that in mind. What is true for knee pain goes as well for depression and for a variety of other very common conditions.

"There are many reasons the elderly may tend to have their depression manifest itself in physical symptoms," says Dr. Lester Krames, director of psychological services at the Hamilton Pain Clinic in Hamilton, Ontario. "Admitting to emotional symptoms of depression may be seen as a threat to independence. It is more acceptable for someone to have physical complaints as they age rather than psychological problems.

"But in general, I would recommend that care givers be sensitive to the complaints raised by the elderly. When these complaints are tied specifically to physical problems, the complaints are probably specific. The patient will say that his knee hurts if his knee hurts.

"But it does pay to become concerned when the complaints become more nonspecific, and when there is a more generalized list of complaints of symptoms. Perhaps someone will say that he just feels lousy all the time, or that everything hurts. This type of thing is more likely to signal some type of mood shift."

If you think that your loved one, whether being taken care of at home or in a care facility, is suffering any of the symptoms discussed in this chapter, you owe it to her to insist that she see a doctor. A confidential chat with a doctor your mom knows and trusts may be all that's required.

If more is required, that doctor will either try some kind of medication or refer her to a psychiatrist. Even if it's a little inconvenient to get her to the psychiatrist, do go. It may change her life.

For more information about depression, contact the office of the Canadian Mental Health Association nearest you. The addresses are in the resource list at the back of this book.

To sum up...

- Depression is very common among the elderly, and may affect up to ten per cent of people in care facilities.

- There are many symptoms of depression, some serious and some not so serious.

- If you think your loved one may be suffering from a serious depression, you owe it to her to get her to seek help.

- Even if she has only a year or two to live, she deserves to have the quality of her life improved for that remaining time.

CHAPTER FOURTEEN
GETTING ACTION ON YOUR COMPLAINTS

No matter how good the care facility your loved one is in, there may still be times when something is not right. No matter how excellent the care, it may lack in certain respects. As with any system, things happen, things go wrong.

Residents' complaints may range from grey meat at dinner to serious abuse and neglect. What should you do?

The first step is listening to your loved one. Let her tell the whole story in her own way, and take notes if you think you won't remember everything. If roommates or other residents are close by and hear your conversation, let them join in. More than one opinion about the matter may be helpful. Only after you have a good grasp of what is really going on can you decide if you can and should do something.

Whatever you do, don't go running to the desk seething and shouting that mom just told me that . . .! This is a sure way to make the situation worse. Instead, use diplomacy. Except in the most serious of cases, you may even want to go home and talk over the situation with the rest of the family before you say or do anything.

If the problem is something very simple, such as a sink that isn't always perfectly sparkling, or the housekeeper who's always rearranging the bottles on the dresser when she dusts, you don't have to make a big production about it. It's usually not necessary to even bring these small complaints to the attention of the staff, and in many cases, is not advisable.

Of course, if your mom seems very upset about a small matter, just talking about it with you will probably help to diffuse her anger. Try not to make light of the complaint, even if it seems petty to you. Remember that sometimes when there is nothing else of importance to do, it's easy to become fixated on one little thing.

Offer your understanding and remind her that the staff is very busy. Don't promise to take care of things, for you may not be able to. Just offer your best reassurances that everything will probably turn out okay. If you've been successful, you probably won't hear the complaint again. If you do, however, it might need a little more consideration.

Many family members prefer not to say anything about such small matters because they don't want to rock the boat. You may also feel that the relationship between your parent, the family and the staff is tenuous, and best not tested.

A public health nurse told me that when her father was in a nursing home, they never brushed his teeth. He only had five teeth, but he wanted to keep them to help anchor his dentures. It was quite a while before he told her about this, because he was embarrassed. But once she knew, rather than complain to the staff, she simply started brushing his teeth for him each time she visited. Everything was a lot simpler this way.

My father never said anything negative to the staff about anything during the six months my mother was in a nursing home, because he was afraid to be viewed as a problem. When he got there each day he always found her slumped over and curled in a corner of the bed, so he always straightened her up and put the pillows around her to prop her up. He also always made sure he visited at dinnertime, so he could feed her and make sure she had plenty of time to eat. He never complained, and I know he was much appreciated by the staff.

You also may choose to say nothing. A good number of the little problems are caused simply by staff shortages, and it's doubtful anything much can be done about them. Nevertheless, the staff at care facilities should value comments from family members, encourage communication between family and staff, for this fosters change where change is needed and allows facilities to improve the quality of care they provide.

Unfortunately, complaints are not always greeted with enthusiasm. And in fact, at some facilities complaining is the last thing you want to do. The tricky part is that you may not know how your complaint will be received until after you've expressed it.

Many people have read stories and seen movies of life in nursing homes, and been horrified by what they read and saw. The sad fact is that not all of these stories are fiction. Conditions are certainly better now than they were twenty years ago, but in some cases the family is right to be wary.

I have heard of cases where the family was upset with the situation their loved one was in, and let it be known over and over. The members of the staff, being human, could take only so much of this. In some instances, certain medical reasons were made up so that the resident could be transferred to another facility—and the family with him. And in a few cases, the anger and frustration of the staff was taken out on the resident. It is probably just this fear of reprisals—physical and verbal abuse or neglect—that keeps so many family members quiet when they see that something is wrong.

But Ryerson School of Nursing professor Kathleen Gates stresses that, even though this fear of reprisal makes people vulnerable, and hesitant sometimes to speak up, nothing will ever change for the better unless family and staff work together in the same direction.

Problems can come when a new resident moves in, and the family is gung-ho about making sure grandma lives out the rest of her life in perfect bliss. Often these unrealistic expectations are fueled by feelings of guilt. They wanted to keep grandma at home, but just couldn't handle it. But they think that they can single-handedly reform the facility so that grandma will be taken care of just as if she was still at home—or maybe even better. Then they can be free of the guilt.

People like this can cause many problems, because they are constantly complaining about the silliest little things. They may even embarrass grandma, who is probably perfectly happy with the place. The only hope for a peaceful end is that they will run out of steam soon, and decide that things aren't so bad after all.

But it must be stressed that every resident, no matter how old or sick, does have the right to a clean, safe and stimulating environment, to good food and a life free of neglect and abuse. One has to keep in mind, however, that whatever biases and prejudices the residents had in their previous life, these may become more pronounced as they get older. So problems may occur when the staff has to deal with them. Not all older people are sweet and dear.

So what should you do if you see that something is *really* wrong?

Most professionals I spoke with felt that if you want to say something, the quiet soft approach is definitely the best. They suggested that you always balance one complaint with at least two compliments. "I love the new window box in the atrium. I'll bet everybody takes turns puttering in it. And mom's hair looks great—it's so nice of you to take the time to see that she's always taken care of. Is there any way you could see that her teeth get brushed a little more often, too? I know she only has four, but she's very fond of them and wants to keep them."

This approach seems to work well with smaller concerns, things that are easy to remedy. Or, as stated before, you may just want to start brushing mom's teeth yourself and not say anything.

Dian Goldstein of Concerned Friends says she had a lot of complaints when her parents were in care facilities, but she was hesitant at first to speak up. Looking back now, she feels she should have handled things differently.

"I think that if I were doing it all over, I would not have put up with the little wrong things at the very beginning. I would have put the pressure on at the very beginning to let them know I was dissatisfied with certain things, and kept up the pressure to let them know I meant business. I think if you start by just pussyfooting around, they hope you'll forget what has happened.

"As each incident occurs your mental and physical strength is kind of progressively sapped away, and it makes it more difficult for you to fight the next battle. As you keep getting put in your place, you start to feel withered and worn out, like a wet leaf, and so find it very difficult to rise to the occasion to fight the next time. Whether this is a conscious effort on the part of the facilities, I don't know. But I believe this is what happens with most people. They get tired of fighting and curl up and just accept the situation."

There are always staff shortages, and if some little jobs can be skipped, things run a lot smoother. So the staff may start with something very small, such as leaving your mother in a housecoat all the time and never dressing her. That saves a bit of time. If you never say anything, then they might try something else, perhaps washing her hair less frequently. That saves more time.

Eventually, if the staff members get away with little things, they may move on to bigger, more important things—such as not giving a few minutes to people who, with a little assistance to and from the washroom and perhaps help in sitting down, are able to use the toilet.

But it takes time to do this, and waiting around for someone to do their thing in the washroom may not be considered a good use of it. So in many facilities diapers are put on everybody, simply because the place does not have the staff to keep running everybody to and from the washroom. A practical solution, perhaps, but not a very dignified one.

So as Ms. Goldstein suggests, you should not keep quiet when you see the little shortcuts starting. Because if you do, chances are good that the bigger, more important things aren't far behind.

I would suggest you feel out the staff first. If they seem cheerful about correcting the first concern, that mother should be fully dressed every day, you're off to a good start. If you're there a lot and keeping an eye on things, they will know you mean business. They will know you're committed to getting the best possible care for your mother. And they will see that she gets it.

If your first suggestion about dressing mother is met with a wince and a comment about how short-staffed they are, then you'll have to use all your judgement, tact and diplomacy when bringing up problems. Or, as suggested earlier, you may have to work around the staff and just correct as many things as you can yourself, or hire a paid companion to come in and do some of them.

If you're complaining about things of a serious nature, you should certainly take some action. In fact, you have an obligation to—not just for your loved one, but also for others living in that care facility who may not have anyone to speak up for them.

Worthy of serious complaints are:

- Problems with meals, such as food that doesn't look or smell right, or some people not being given enough time to eat.

- Unsafe conditions, such as emergency doors chained shut, or small objects in the hallways that people could trip on.

- Signs of neglect, such as bruises or bedsores.

"If you have concerns or grievances about the care your relative is getting in a care facility, speak up," insists Dr. Yoel Isenberg. "Some institutions have ombudsmen, and there should be a patient advisory committee or residents' council. A family advisory committee has the means for relatives to have input and to obtain clarification, hopefully to their satisfaction, regarding physicians.

"But remember that institutions do have real budgetary constraints and cannot always provide the kind of one-on-one care that ideally you would want your loved one to have. It is important to bring up your concern, however, and see if it can be resolved."

If everything cannot be worked out to your satisfaction, what can you do to make sure that your loved one gets the best possible care given the circumstances? Even if the place she's in is less than ideal, you may not want to move her because the trauma of the move could be worse.

Always start by discussing her care with the nursing staff and the physician. There should also be an administrative pathway for you to pass along your concerns. That could be through a social worker, an ombudsman or other representative of the administration. If you see something that just doesn't look right or feel right, pursue it.

My father never said anything to anyone at the nursing home because he was afraid to make waves. And such fears are realistic, for there's no guarantee about how someone will respond. You can't be sure the staff won't perceive somebody as a troublemaker, and cause more problems for the resident in the long run.

Dr. Isenberg suggests that you raise concerns in a tactful manner and show that you're looking for a realistic resolution, rather than merely airing complaints. And there are ways of raising issues that are more likely to lead to a positive resolution.

For example, Dr. D. William Molloy suggests that you ask to attend the staff meetings that are held to assess each resident's care. These meetings, which are called different things in different facilities, are attended by everyone who is responsible for care: at least one doctor, the head nurse or other nurses, the social worker, and perhaps the recreation director and the dietitian.

Such meetings are an excellent way not only to find out what is really going on with your relative and her care, but also a perfect opportunity to bring up concerns and complaints. It's a calm forum for calm discussion, rather than a confrontation with one person who may react badly to what you have to say.

You probably won't be told when these meetings are, so you will have to ask. If nobody will tell you, ask louder. The staff cannot shut you out of these meetings. The trick is finding out when they are so you can be there. Don't hesitate to go to administration if the staff refuses to give you this information, although you'll find that in most cases, you will be welcomed. The staff likes to know that you care enough to make a special trip to attend.

If there's something you want to talk about, Dr. Molloy recommends that you tell the staff ahead of time, so that everyone you need in the discussion will be at the meeting. If you want particularly to discuss, for example, why your mother is put into diapers when you know she can go to the washroom by herself if only someone would help her get there, you should ask in advance that a particular doctor and the head nurse be present at the meeting you'll be attending. You should listen carefully to everything they say about your mother, and perhaps take notes.

After everyone has given his or her view of your mother's current situation, you are free to add comments and questions. You may want to start out with a few compliments—how clean everything always is, for instance—and then tactfully raise your concerns.

When my father and I attended a meeting like this for my mother, our main worry was that she was losing weight so rapidly. We requested that the dietitian be there, and also her general doctor. When we brought the subject up, they didn't seem terribly concerned, saying that this happens to most people with her problem. But we told them that *we* were terribly concerned, and couldn't they please do something? They started her on supplemental feeding immediately.

Did they neglect to do this sooner because they were just so used to seeing people waste away to nothing, or did they think she wouldn't last as long anyway and wanted to save a little money? It doesn't matter why. All that matters is that she was given the supplemental feeding, and this probably made her final months a little better.

Joan Fussell of Concerned Friends suggests you be wary when you attend a staff meeting. She said that sometimes the meeting is "loaded" with a lot of people who may put up a united front against you. You should try to take someone with you, so you don't have to face them all alone.

She also recommends that you go to the meeting prepared with notes and a clear mind about the complaints and questions you want the professionals to address. After the meeting, you should write to the administrator. Include the outline of your concerns, list any commitments made by the staff, and mention any concerns that were not satisfactorily taken care of at the meeting.

If this method does not eventually resolve your concerns, then you will have to take further action. Concerned Friends recommend you do the following when you have serious complaints:[1]

Complaints can be made by phone or by letter. All complaints made by phone should be followed up with a letter. A good letter of complaint should include:

- the name of the institution about which you are complaining

- the name of the resident about whom you are concerned

- your name and your relationship to the resident

- a concise summary of your concern and complaints

- a request for a response in writing

- a request that your complaint be handled in a confidential manner, if you wish

"If these measures fail to bring about a satisfactory improvement in the conditions," Ms. Fussell adds, "then families should not hesitate to go to the branch of government that funds and oversees that type of institution."

The resource list at the end of the book has the addresses and phone numbers of people in the federal and provincial governments ultimately responsible for care facilities. If you have serious problems you cannot get solved at the facility, they want to know about them. Write them, including all of the information listed above, and send a copy of your letter to the administrator of the care facility in question.

Another way relatives can try to have input at a care facility is by participating in the residents' council. Many councils get a lot of important things done on behalf of the residents, and many changes are due to this action. And it's the changes that the residents themselves want that are ultimately the most valuable, both to current and future residents.

Anything you can do to help your loved one eventually will help all the other people who will spend time in that same facility. Never be afraid to take action on serious problems.

---

[1]Reprinted with permission from Concerned Friends from their brochure "Avenues of Complaint Regarding the Welfare of Ontario Citizens in Care Facilities"

The following was prepared by Dian Goldstein for her course on Seniors Studies at Ryerson Polytechnical Institute in Toronto. She is pleased to share her wisdom in this book.

How to get things done[1]

1. Believe in yourself or your group. Believe that you have power. Recognize that you have as much understanding of the situation as any authority figure.

2. Know what your objective is. What do you want to achieve? Be very clear and focussed on your goal. Write it down. Does it make sense when you talk about it? If you want people to listen, you must understand the situation completely.

3. Ask questions of everyone. Where, when, how, why, and especially who. Discuss your issues with experts in the field.

4. Learn all you can about the situation by asking questions. What is the mandate? What are the operating principles? Read to get information— from government documents, newsletters, annual reports, journals, daily newspapers, magazines, brochures, program reports, planning documents and copies of legislation.

5. Go and visit people. Identify the persons and agencies that can make the decisions needed to satisfy your needs. Find a reason to go to other groups that may have like interests, and read their mandates. You may find helpful people to network with; gain their support.

6. Be proud to be a consumer. After all, you do pay for the services provided to you. Be proud to be a volunteer. People in power often act in a condescending manner toward volunteers. Don't let them. Be proud of your accomplishments and what you're striving for.

7. Write—write—write. Your ideas, views, experiences and opinions *are* important. Share them with government, people with similar interests, groups with like causes, the newspapers, newsletters, and so on. Don't forget thank-you's and suggestions. Write about good things and things you would like to change, and suggest how you think it might be done.

8. Take risks. Don't be afraid to try something new. If you are prepared, you will make *some* impact. Advocacy efforts work a little at a time.

---

[1] Prepared by and reprinted with permission from Dian Goldstein from her course on Seniors Studies at Ryerson Polytechnical Institute in Toronto.

9. Tell other people what you are doing. Share information, particularly if you achieve success. Accept help from others. You can't expect to know everything and do everything by yourself.

10. Remember—what you do counts. It can help others in the future. If you don't choose to do something, someone else will choose for you.

How to complain[1]

1. Get the necessary support in the form of letters from experts which show *concrete data* or explanations. Remember, your feelings and subjective experiences are not enough.

2. Find out who makes the decisions. Who has the power? Write to them. Phone them.

3. Present cases or ideas verbally and in writing to the person in power. Keep copies of all of your letters and any responses you get.

4. Use existing structures within the line of command. Begin at the lowest level and move up the hierarchy if you still don't have satisfaction.

5. Remember: Be fearless. Don't be intimidated. Focus on what you can do.

6. Persist—issues are often lost because someone gave up. Expect someone to say no at the start, but don't accept it as the final word. Don't let others laugh at you or put you down—be thick-skinned. And really listen to what people say to you and ask them why? or why not? Don't just accept their platitudes and give up.

To sum up...

- Really listen to what your loved one has to say about the facility and any complaints she may have. Take notes to document problems.

- If her complaints are small, it's probably easier to do something about them yourself than constantly bother the staff.

- If the problems are serious, you must take action. Everyone, no matter how old or sick, has a right to good basic care and respect, and a life free from neglect and abuse.

- There are several avenues of complaint, and they range from a little chat with a nurse to calling TV stations and newspapers. Always start with the minimum, and move up the ladder only if you are absolutely forced to.

---

[1] Prepared by and reprinted with permission from Dian Goldstein from her course on Seniors Studies at Ryerson Polytechnical Institute in Toronto.

- But if conditions are deplorable, you are sure of your facts, and you are forced to take action, do it right. Call your MP, and call the media.

- In the resource list at the back of the book are addresses and phone numbers of the people in government who are ultimately responsible for care facilities. If you cannot get satisfaction at the facility, contact them. That's what they're there for.

- Concerned Friends of Ontario Citizens in Care Facilities is a volunteer, nonprofit organization that advocates on behalf of institutionalized citizens. They recognize the need for increased community support, improved quality of care for institutionalized residents, and constructive changes to statutes governing long-term-care facilities. They are doing wonderful work to improve the lot of all people who need care. If you would like to start a similar group in your area, please contact them for more information at Box 1054, Station Q, Toronto, Ontario M4T 2P2.

CHAPTER FIFTEEN

MONEY MEANS CHOICES

Only about one in ten of us will be able to carry our pre-retirement lifestyle into retirement. Socio-economic level has very little bearing on this ominous situation.

The bulk of retirement income comes from the government, former-employer pension plans, private and personal sources. We can no longer depend on government pensions—one example is the old-age security clawback. Some experts suggest that the Canada Pension Plan will not be able to continue giving out current benefits in the future, and so this money may not be available to baby boomers when they reach retirement age.

Many employees have been restricted in the amount of money they can place in their RRSP because of company pension contributions. By law, in most provinces a surviving spouse receives sixty per cent of the deceased spouse's company pension. And most pensions are not indexed to offset the ravages of inflation.

I asked Dale Ennis, publisher of *Canadian MoneySaver*, a personal-finance magazine, what this situation will mean to Canadians who want not only to retire to their pre-retirement lifestyle, but who want to be sure they have enough set aside to cover the possibility of their becoming ill or incapacitated. Because as much as we would like to think that we will just go to bed perfectly healthy one night and die peacefully in our sleep, the fact is that many of us will need care of one kind or another in our later years. And unfortunately, good care costs money.

"The onus is on each individual to begin financial planning as early as possible, in order to build a personal income source for the future," Mr. Ennis says. "Starting to plan for retirement earlier can significantly improve an individual's financial picture."

He suggests you sit down right now and see what the future may hold for you. By using copies of The Seniors' Guide to Federal Programs and Services, and information on your provincial programs—see the resource list in the back of the book for ordering these free booklets—you can gain some insight into what will be available to you when you retire.

For company-pension data, speak to your payroll clerk or the appropriate administrator. Determine exactly what your pension will be and what your spouse would get if you died.

"Armed with this information," Mr. Ennis says, "you should be in a realistic position to calculate your retirement income. Advanced planning is necessary, particularly financial planning, because financial status has a major impact on all aspects of our well-being."

If you are that fortunate one in ten, you may not need a budget to determine your financial position. But a budget gives you a clear picture of your expenses. It will show you how much money you can "pay" yourself before you begin taking care of regular expenses and debts.

Mr. Ennis suggests you begin by setting aside a comfortable portion of your monthly funds for personal investing, and increase this amount when you can.

"It is important that you become your own money expert. You have to be able to understand your investments and know where your money goes."

There are many knowledgeable advisors who can assist you, but you have to know your own finances before you invest. As you learn more about your personal position, assets and income, your confidence will increase and you will sleep better at night, knowing that you're prepared for the future, no matter what happens.

For a free copy of *Canadian MoneySaver*, which explains money and investing in simple, easy-to-understand terms, just write to Box 370, Bath, Ontario K0H 1G0, or phone (613) 352-7448.

Jury Kopach, president of Murray Axmith Retirement Services Inc. and publisher of *The Retirement Letter*, is a retirement planner whose main job is providing retirement planning services to corporations for their employees. For more information, contact him at 130 Bloor St. West, Suite 802, Toronto, Ontario M5S 1N5, or phone (416) 961-0632.

I asked him about the changes people have to go through as they age, and why planning for retirement is so important.

"I think it's a fact," he responds, "that people handle change very poorly, simply because they don't prepare themselves for it. We tend to structure our lives according to a plan, and that plan has a blueprint. Historically that basically is school, followed by work or a job, followed by marriage, followed by kids, buying your house, the promotion and then retirement.

"Virtually that's where the plan ends, and during that period we've got all sorts of support structures. We have counsellors at work, teachers at school, and so on."

Mr. Kopach believes that the main problem for most people is that we have no plan past retirement, even though we now live twenty, thirty or even forty years in retirement. And the second problem is that we don't really seek to develop new support systems once we retire.

So when people retire, they like the change in one way, because now they have a lot of freedom, but in another way they are very much afraid of it.

People seldom if ever plan for becoming dependent and perhaps having to go into a nursing home. They just refuse to think about it—out of mind, out of sight. The attitude is—like the prospect of a heart attack or a stroke—"it will never happen to me."

People worry about a place in Florida rather than a nursing home. It's one of the unpleasant things in life that we simply don't want to deal with. So consequently not too many people plan for it. Most people think they will be perfectly well until they die.

Mr. Kopach thinks that many people feel they are not going to die at all, that they'll live forever. "Death is so foreign to them. But I think that stems from the fact that we have changed our family unit. The family unit no longer includes grandparents. Grandparents are just out there somewhere, and when they get sick or need nursing care, children don't see them—and so we really have no experience in dealing with illness as a family unit. We don't have the bond.

"We have isolated ourselves, and we've created environments for ourselves, and therefore we really have trouble dealing with death because not only do we not see it in other people, we don't plan for it ourselves. But everybody's been telling us it's good to be independent. Well, I think ultimately it works against us.

"The baby boomers are going to be in really big trouble because they are the most independent of all. My best advice for them is essentially to become more dependent as they get older, particularly if they're single. I see it starting to happen. A good example is two single people buying a home together once they retire. Their bonds are not so much the housing, it's the taking care of each other.

"As time goes by there are going to be a lot more people who are all alone. But there's nothing like another human being, as opposed to an institution, to take care of you—and I think that's where a lot of people should be looking, particularly those who are single.

"But I think the independence issue is a very important one. We are taught to be independent, but ultimately we have to be dependent on someone else, whether it's physically or monetarily or something other than that.

"Historically we've been dependent on our families. But I think the dependency issue has now unfortunately been focussed on the governments. We are dependent on governments and governments are broke and governments are faced with humanless entities, and that's the tragedy of the whole thing. We are dependent on governments to build homes, we are dependent on governments for advice, we're dependent on governments period. I think the objective should be that people

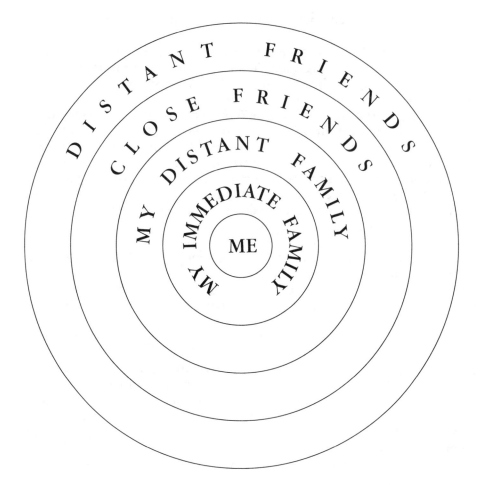

going into retirement—particularly those who are single—should try to build bonds with other people."

Mr. Kopach shared the above illustration with me for the book. In this illustration, picture yourself as the dot in the centre. You are the centre of your own universe. Everything revolves around you. Surrounding that dot is a circle that includes your closest family—your spouse, your children, your parents. Surrounding that are the distant family members, your aunts, uncles and so on. Outside of that are your close friends, and the last outer circle around that includes your distant friends.

As you go into retirement, your closest family either dies or moves away or becomes distant from you. So the whole idea is to replace that family with the next circle, the distant family, so that you start bringing people in closer to you. Then you start bringing people in from the close friends, then the distant friends. The idea is to bring each circle closer as you age, to build an emotional and physical support network for yourself.

Mr. Kopach believes that people want change, but they are afraid of it—so they don't plan for it. And if they do plan for change they only plan for *positive* change and not *negative* change. People simply don't ask themselves enough questions of the "what if" type.

For example, if my parents or one of my parents became ill at retirement would I be able to take them into my home? That involves a lot of questions—moral questions, financial questions, ethical questions and so forth. People simply refuse to ask themselves these questions. What if my spouse became ill? What would I do? Or what if I were left alone? What would happen?

In other words, there simply aren't enough questions like these being asked. Certainly people hear about nursing homes and illness. But it's like a smoker. A smoker hears all that bad news out there that if he continues to smoke he's going to get cancer and his risk of heart attack will go up, but he simply refuses to listen, primarily because he feels it will never happen to him.

People have not had the luxury or the experience of looking at a whole generation of individuals who will be in retirement a quarter to a third of their lives. So there is nothing out there that we can look back at and say, "See, this generation did it successfully, so we should be doing it the same way."

We just don't have that luxury. We've never lived as long and never retired as early. So we don't have the luxury of a previous blueprint. And that's why the generation entering retirement now is really at the forefront of something very new.

So what good advice does Mr. Kopach have to offer us? Well, essentially the advice is to start thinking for ourselves rather than relying on others to take the responsibility for our lives. Don't put it all off on the government or your employer, or perhaps even your family. You're the one living the rest of your life, so you're responsible for it. And that includes the good and the bad.

What about the baby boomers who are now starting to see their parents retire? Mr. Kopach believes that their parents are probably luckier, as they are part of the wealthiest generation to have ever experienced retirement. He doubts very much that the baby boomers in retirement will be as well off as their parents.

Baby boomers must realize that one-quarter of the population will be sixty-five or older at the same time they are. That will cause tremendous stress on things we take for granted now, such as provincial health insurance, nursing homes—all the things we now simply take for granted because they're there.

But an economic or tax base in Canada to support what we have right now, what the current retired generation has now, simply won't be there. So boomers are looking at an even more difficult situation than their parents are. And that's why they should be planning much earlier. And that's why that baby boom generation has to ask itself the "what if" questions—especially taking into account that the divorce rate is forty per cent and many of them will be single.

Mr. Kopach stresses that he's not a doom-and-gloomer, but he is a realist. If you simply look at what's going on in Canada, you'll see that our birthrate is declining and our average age is increasing. Unless we experience huge population increases due to immigration, there won't be any change. Our tax base is shrinking. Canada Pension Plan is underfunded and virtually broke. There won't be enough there to pay the baby boomers. And now more and more people are freelancing and working part-time, so they won't have company pensions.

We should look far enough into the future to ask ourselves questions like: what if the government doesn't have any money when I reach retirement? We should be putting away at least five to ten per cent of our salary every year. If not, we are going to be in trouble. The boomers are going to experience a lower standard of living than the present generation.

I asked Mr. Kopach how he feels this situation will affect the care situation in Canada.

"I think our society will simply have to change. The home-care industry now basically depends on government support. Even the private homes get government support, and look at how much they are charging—phenomenal amounts of money. Now people are selling their homes, the largest part of their assets, and they are using that as capital to move into retirement homes. But twenty-five years down the road, the baby boomers will have moved into retirement. When they try to sell their homes to raise some money, there will be fewer people buying, and so the value of homes will go down.

"The population won't have the purchasing power and the capital assets needed to buy their way into the present nursing homes. Either you are going to have deterioration in care or you're going to have a different social structure where essentially parents will have to move in with their children and children will have to become guardians and health-care givers whether they like it or not. It will not be the 'me' generation anymore, it will be a dependent generation.

"That's why I'm saying that society is going to have to change. And my advice is don't look to the government for help because there are too many people retiring right now thinking the government's going to take care of them. And the government has planted this attitude in people—

'Don't worry about retirement, you will be taken care of.' North American governments have done that.

"The attitude is that someone's going to take care of you, because we've been reared on that type of a culture. Your family takes care of you, the school takes care of you, the employer takes care of you. But when you're retired and you have a problem, who do you run to? The worst thing that I see is that people who are retiring do not think for themselves."

I asked Mr. Kopach what he feels are the three most important questions people should be asking themselves now.

"Well, the first question is, 'Can I afford retirement?' The second most important question is the financial issue. You need roughly seventy-five per cent of your normal income to maintain the same standard of living after you retire. That's a rule of thumb. Most people's pensions will add up to between seventy and seventy-five per cent. But many people's idea of retirement is Club Med, and if it's a Club Med retirement they want, then they are going to need 110 per cent. So it depends on what your objective is.

"The third question is basically, 'What are the support mechanisms I need to put into place before I retire to maintain the same standard of living I have now?' And people never ask that. People don't build the supporting mechanisms because they have had them built for them all their lives.

"One supporting mechanism is the emotional one—that if I need help, if I'm ill and need help, who do I go to? Who do I tell that I'm sick? The standard in our society is that you've got to be healthy, otherwise you're useless. Who do I go to? This is a very critical point, which I find people have a great deal of difficulty with."

Mr. Kopach also feels that people need to prepare a book that essentially spells out what they want in case of an accident or illness. It should contain lists of what you need and what you want. And this book should be updated, just like a will, every five years, should be handled just like a will or a power of attorney. Lawyers should recommend something like this to people when they come in to have their wills made or updated.

Banks should have forms or booklets or pamphlets that would help people to ask themselves the questions. Of course, if a person really doesn't want to think about the future, there is nothing you can do for her. But at least if she is confronted with it, she will ask herself the questions and perhaps do something about them.

We must consider the issues of growing old and growing helpless in terms of our family unit. Because we don't have grandmothers and grandfathers living with us any longer, we don't see what happens. Children and even adults don't see what happens in old age. And if you don't see it and if you don't understand it, you don't think about it—and therefore you don't react to it. So much of the plight of the elderly is not their fault. It's a result of the way we've structured our family units and our society. You can't change this. Money is a very serious concern here, because perhaps twenty-five years from now, only if you have money will you have choices as far as the care situation goes.

And right now or in the very near future, if you don't have a lot of money you won't have much choice—you'll have to keep the elderly and ill person at home and somebody will have to stay at home with him, because you won't be able to afford a private nurse. So if you don't have money you'll be stuck and you won't have any choice. Money is a very big factor, but another equally big factor is attitude. Both are very important.

People must plan and people must make the necessary commitment. They have to do the research, they have to ask themselves the right questions, they have to set money aside. They have to essentially look at the alternatives. Things have worked out very well for the people who have done this, whether they've become ill or not. When people don't ask themselves those questions and leave the responsibility to someone else or the government, that's where you see the tragedies.

If your elderly widowed mother comes to you and asks if she can move in, what should you do? The first step is to consider the cost and available support services in your community. Have a good look at your budget. Can you afford another mouth to feed? Extra medical costs? Only after you have considered these things can you have an intelligent discussion about it with your family.

But what if your mother comes to you and asks whether she can live with you, and you know you can't afford it, or you simply don't want her there? You should sit down with mother and discuss it with her. Tell her that you've looked around, and this is what you've come up with, and that you want to sit down and make a rational decision together.

So it's not only the older people who have to ask "what if." When tragedy strikes, everyone's under stress, everyone's emotionally differ-ent in terms of what their reaction might be, and the decisions are made in short order without the necessary information—and that's when a lot of mistakes happen.

That's when people say to themselves, "I wish I had known." But all it takes is a few hours of your time five years before retirement or even at retirement to start doing that research, because people who have done it have been very successful. When illness hits, the preparation makes all the difference.

Making a simple budget is part of the planning. If people can see ahead of time how much extra money they will have, that would be ideal. Before they have a budget, most people would say that they couldn't possibly scrape together another dime. Most people would say it was impossible, they don't have anything in the bank, they couldn't save a penny, they need every cent just to live. But if you ask the right questions, most people can find some extra money. So when tragedy strikes, most people are able either to help mother to stay in her own home with extra money for cabs and delivery services, or to take her in, or to find her a nice place to live where she gets good care.

Let's consider a scenario where your elderly mother breaks her hip, and you know she won't be able to stay in her home alone once she gets out of the hospital. You'd love to take her in, but you know that will mean a lot of extra expenses.

You want to make things nice for her, so you fix up the spare room, buy a comfortable new bed for her, a walker or wheelchair, maybe an elevation device on the stairway, probably some maid service, nursing care when needed, maybe even an occasional paid companion. But you generally only have nineteen dollars left at the end of every month after your own expenses. How can you reconcile a situation like that?

It can be very difficult if you haven't planned ahead. If you've had the foresight to draw up a budget and start a savings plan, you'll probably be in good shape. Most people can live on ninety-five per cent of what they're taking in. If you can start saving five per cent of your income every month, and you compound that, it grows to unbelievable amounts very quickly. You just need the self-discipline to put away the money each and every month. It's taking a portion of your income right off the top and calling it "paying yourself for the future."

Open a special account for this money, so that it is kept separate. Call it your retirement fund, or call it whatever you want, but keep this money set aside for that specific purpose. You might have to use it to take in your mother—it will depend on the situations that come up—but at least you will have some money available.

In addition to that special fund, you should also be paying yourself for the future—your own pension fund. Ideally it would be ten per cent of your salary, but if you can only afford three per cent, then fine.

But what if the situation with your mother happens before you've done anything? What if you have no savings at all? Mother needs you now, and you feel you can't help her.

You love your mother, and of course you want to give her the very best available. You wish you could afford to put her in a $3000-a-month home where she will have the best of everything, but you know you can't. If you haven't set anything aside and haven't planned ahead, don't feel guilty. Like most people, you just didn't think anything would ever happen. And if nothing else, this experience will certainly get you planning your own retirement and financial future in a hurry!

There's no easy answer to a situation like this, where there is no

money for an emergency situation. It may be a case of borrowing money
or going into debt, or selling some assets. You may have a boat or a
cottage that you could sell, or perhaps stocks or bonds. If you don't have
assets, then you borrow. If you have no assets and you have no credit
rating, then you can't help your mother financially. You may be able to
help her emotionally and in other ways, but you won't be able to help her
financially. The other option is that you may have to take her in and
provide the services she needs, such as nursing, yourself.

For an elderly couple with no children and no savings, the situation
can be very bleak. Imagine a couple who live in an apartment, and so
have no major assets such as a house. The husband gets Alzheimer's, and
although the wife does her best to take care of him, eventually he has to
go into a nursing home. The wife is in fine health, but she's seventy-five
and obviously can't get a job. Now all of a sudden she's responsible for
the rent and other expenses all by herself, because her husband's money
is going to the home.

Mr. Kopach recommends that anyone who finds herself in a situation like this must first learn to handle finances. She should go and see a
qualified financial planner to sort things out and take a careful look at
her situation. She shouldn't attempt to sort things out herself. The
financial planner should be a qualified one, who is independent and
gives advice for a fee. There are a lot of people out there who give advice
by selling a product; it's easier in the long run and better to pay money
for advice.

The planner will help her take a look at her net worth and decide if
she has any assets she could sell to pay for her standard of living—that is,
if there isn't enough income otherwise. Since her husband has become
ill, he may have an insurance policy that could take care of him. The
financial advisor will help her find out.

Mr. Kopach supplied the budget sheet at the end of this chapter. You
might want to do a little planning this evening. This budget will show
you clearly if there is no extra money available for a private retirement
fund after your expenses. But there are many things you can do. Cut
your debt, trim your expenses. Start setting aside just five per cent of
your income somehow. You'll thank yourself tomorrow.

To sum up . . .

- Emergencies can happen in a minute, so you have to be ready.

- You cannot depend on anyone else to help you.

- Only if you have some money do you have choices.

Net Worth Statement

WHAT YOU OWN

CASH	
Savings Accounts	
Chequing Accounts . .	
Other	
TOTAL	

INVESTMENTS	
Bonds	
Stocks	
Mutual Funds	
Life Insce CSV	
RRSP's	
Other	
Company Pension . . .	
TOTAL	

REAL ESTATE	
Residence	
Other	
TOTAL	

PERSONAL PPTY	
Automobiles	
Furniture	
Appliances	
Jewellery	
Recreation Vehicles . .	
TOTAL	

TOTAL OWNED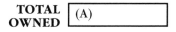

WHAT YOU OWE

CURRENT BILLS	
Charge Accounts	
Medical & Dental	
Other	
. . . .	
. . . .	
. . . .	
. . . .	
TOTAL	

DEBTS	
Charge Accounts	
Personal Loans	
Insurance Loans	
Mortgages	
Installment Loans	
Other	
. . . .	
TOTAL	

TOTAL OWED

TOTAL OWNED	(A)
TOTAL OWED	(B)
YOUR NET WORTH	(C)

Budget Planner

Monthly Take Home Pay

Wages / Salary	
Wages / Salary	
Family Allowance Pension	
Other Regular Monthly Income	
TOTAL MONTHLY TAKE-HOME INCOME	

Monthly Budget

Monthly Savings	Emergency Fund	
	TOTAL MONTHLY SAVINGS Line 1	

Monthly Living Expenses	Food (plus other grocery store items)		
	Housing	1st Mortgage or Rent	
		2nd Mortgage	
	Utilities (total from box "A" on next page)		
	Household Incidentals		
	Transportation	Gasoline	
		Bus Fares	
		Parking	
	Personal Allowances & Recreation (total from box B on next page)		
	Other (child support, alimony, child care, household help, etc.)		
	Monthly Requirement for Irregular and Annual Expenses (total from Box "C" on next page)		
	TOTAL MONTHLY LIVING EXPENSES Line 2		

Monthly Credit Payments		
	TOTAL MONTHLY CREDIT PAYMENTS Line 3	

TOTAL MONTHLY BUDGET	(Add Line 1, Line 2, and Line 3)	

Budget Planner (cont'd)

Budget Details

Transfer the totals from boxes A, B, and C to the shaded boxes in the Monthly Budget on the previous page

A MONTHLY UTILITIES

Power		
Water / Sewage / Waste		
Telephone		
	Long Distance	
Natural Gas		
Cable TV / Pay TV		
TOTAL MONTHLY UTILITIES		

B MONTHLY AMOUNTS FOR PERSONAL ALLOWANCES AND RECREATION

Personal Allowances (monthly amounts for each family member)		
Family Recreation		
TOTAL MONTHLY PERSONAL ALLOWANCE AND RECREATION		

Scribble Space

C IRREGULAR AND ANNUAL EXPENSES

(All figures in this box should be annual amounts)

Clothing (annual amount for each member)		
Insurance (if you pay directly)	Vehicles	
	Life	
	Property	
	Other	
Medication and Medical Fees		
Dental and Optical		
Education	Tuition	
	Supplies	
Taxes (if you pay directly)	Property	
	Income	
Licences	Vehicles	
	Other	
Maintenance	Vehicles	
	Home & Garden	
	Furnishings	
Gifts and Festivities	Christmas	
	Other	
Contributions and Donations		
Memberships and Season Tickets		
Other (Subscriptions, and planned purchases for next year)		
TOTAL IRREGULAR AND ANNUAL EXPENSES		

↓ divide by 12 ↓

MONTHLY REQUIREMENT FOR IRREGULAR/ANNUAL EXPENSE	

CHAPTER SIXTEEN

HELPING THE DISABLED STAY IN THEIR HOMES

Just like the elderly, most disabled people want to stay in their own homes until they are absolutely forced to move into a care facility. To achieve this end, they need pretty much the same things as the elderly.

But in addition to the universal needs for help with cleaning the house, doing the shopping and finding transportation, many disabled people also need attendant care, which takes care of personal needs, such as getting in and out of bed, bathing, eating, and so on. Exactly what is needed varies with the disability. Some people need very little help, others need help with almost everything.

Unfortunately, no matter where you live, there is never enough attendant care. You'll probably be able to get some, but it's seldom that you can get as much as you really need, and when you need it. This is another area the government will have to look into for health-care reform.

People who have enough money can hire attendants from private companies to meet their needs, but unfortunately, most disabled people do not have much money. Many are unable to work, and so must live on small pensions, which are never enough. Even if someone can work, the medications, appliances and extra help that may be needed all take a big chunk out of a salary.

But with ongoing support from family, friends and neighbours, many people can manage just fine at home even if money is tight. Often two or more disabled people set up housekeeping together, sometimes with others who are not disabled, so that each can help take care of the others. This helps a lot of people remain independent. Many professionals feel that these small group homes are the way of the future. What is needed is more money to be made available for the purchase and outfitting of these homes, and for more people to be accepting of them in their neighbourhoods.

One excellent group I came across is the Cheshire Homes Foundation Canada Inc. They work with concerned citizens to provide services in housing, including specially adapted small group homes, accessible units in regular apartment buildings, and outreach services in people's own homes. They have a variety of services and will gladly send you information. Contact them at 40 Orchard View Blvd., Suite 211, Toronto, Ontario M4R 1B9, or phone (416) 487-0443.

Some disabled people just cannot make it on their own, or just cannot find enough help to enable them to stay at home, and so they have to move into care facilities. Sometimes a young disabled person may be the only one in a nursing home where everyone else is over eighty, and this can be very distressing.

"Young handicapped people often get placed in long-term facilities because there is nothing else," says Nancy Stone, president of the Ontario Association for Community Living. "In these facilities there is no programming for the young people—they just degenerate. There has to be a better way. The solution has to be innovative. Young people have a lot to contribute, no matter how disabled they may be, and we have to pay attention to this contribution."

Beth Chambers, director of Individual and Family Services for the Ontario Division of the Multiple Sclerosis Society of Canada says: "We definitely need more health outreach programs. We also need extended hours for homemaking services. Home care does not always meet the needs of clients, so they must pay to hire a private company. Many clients fall through the cracks."

Some disabled people from rural areas have to move to a big city in order to get the attendant and home care they need in order to remain independent. But in some areas, although there may be fewer services, there are fewer disabled people who need them. So the level of care can be very good.

Moving can sometimes be a bad idea. Although the disabled person may indeed be able to live more independently and get better home care in a larger city, in order to do this he may have to leave behind family and friends. Most professionals I spoke with about this feel that it's usually better to stay close to your family, who can provide help and support of a kind unavailable anywhere else.

Getting help

Accessing the services to help your disabled loved one remain home and independent is not always easy. If something is missing from her life, try calling some of the names in the resource list at the back of the book—the occupational therapy associations may be a good place to start.

Be very specific about what you need. If she needs transportation to the university on Tuesdays, ask specifically for that. If she needs help getting in and out of bed and getting dressed, say that. The more specific you can be, the easier it will be for them to direct you to the right people.

People disabled by multiple sclerosis present unique problems. "Even if you find exactly the right people to help you," says Ms.

Chambers, "quite often symptoms flare up and then subside, so services are required for a period of time, and then not needed. It is often difficult for a person to obtain services again and they must go through a long-drawn-out process of applying again.

"Those very disabled by diseases like multiple sclerosis are often not accepted by various attendant-care services as it is assumed that their condition will deteriorate and necessitate additional care. Many MS clients remain on waiting lists for a very long time."

How well the needs of disabled people are being met in care facilities is directly related to the individual setting and the support provided by the family and volunteers. Most activities and routines in a facility are tailored to older people, and so a thirty-year-old disabled person may have a lot of difficulty. There is a need for a more homelike atmosphere, decision-making related to routines, independence and interaction with the community and outside world. A young person who never spends time with anyone but mentally impaired eighty-year-olds will lead a very deprived life.

The severely disabled will require assistance with all aspects of daily living, and may have limited or no method of communication. Volunteers and family play a large role in ensuring an adequate quality of life.

"There is no easy answer to help make life as good as possible," Ms. Chambers continues. "It is dependent on a person's individual needs. The family should develop a working relationship with the help organizations, which can direct the client to specialized and government programs. It is difficult for the clients not to feel all alone and to feel that they are fighting for their rights all the time."

One of the best things you can do is to contact the national and provincial chapters of organizations for people with your loved one's particular disability. (Many of these are listed in the resource list. They can direct you to others.) These organizations do a lot more than just offer literature that explains the problems associated with each disability.

For example, the purpose of the Ontario Division Individual and Family Services Department is to offer support to the person with multiple sclerosis and his family, and to assist in retaining or regaining a realistic degree of independence and self-determination.

This department's programs and services include:

- information on MS and referral to appropriate community resources

- support and consultation involving the MS person, family members and local community support services

- education on MS for persons with MS, family members and health professionals

- equipment provision and special assistance where appropriate and related to need for persons with MS

- community groups and programs such as self-help groups, swimming and recreation programs, transportation and social events

- special action related to issues to improve the quality of life of all persons with MS, and individual advocacy

Sudden disabilities

"There is a great deal that can be done to assist people in staying in their homes after a sudden disability," said Barbara Baptiste, president and director of Toronto's Rehabilitation Management, Inc. "One of the things that we do is provide an analysis of all of the long-term needs and care, and the related costs, following disability. Because of this we are very aware of what devices are needed and where support services are required.

"Help can range from simple changes, which include a control of the environment (lighting, heating), accessibility to emergency services (fire, police, ambulance), the provision of special bathing and toileting devices and utilization of hospital beds. The needs for the physically disabled vary substantially with the disability. Those individuals who are bound to a wheelchair, for example, also require changes in the accessibility of cupboards and the like, which they have to be able to reach.

"Individuals who have disabilities should have the situation assessed by qualified rehabilitation specialists who have the knowledge and experience to look at the entire environment and implement the necessary changes. The family and friends of disabled persons need to insist on comprehensive, quality services and not be satisfied when people tell them those services are not available. If someone tells you this, ask someone else. Keep looking. You'll find help.

"If someone has to move into a care facility, the family must serve as a strong advocate for the disabled individual to ensure that he gets the necessary care. People who have no families are often left at the discretion of the institutional care providers. The majority of people who work in care facilities wish to provide the highest quality care, but are often limited in the approach they can take or the amount of assistance they can give to an individual.

"Care facilities must become more responsive to a disabled resident's individual needs, and they can do this by really listening to the disabled individuals," Ms. Baptiste continues. "They will tell you the most about what can and what needs to be done. I think that for far too long professionals have been telling the disabled persons what they should be doing rather than listening to them. Disabled people are often quite capable of outlining their needs. A consistent constellation of requests from a group should alert everyone to the fact that those needs must be addressed.

"In addition, care facilities will only improve to the extent that the care providers in them continue to open themselves up to bold moves and decisions. They need to realize that perhaps their way of providing service requires alternative strategies, and they need to remain flexible to new ideas and the concept of change."

Ms. Baptiste recommends that you take along a skilled professional if you are looking at care facilities for a disabled relative, someone who will know which questions to ask and which issues to address. She feels that it's best to get someone involved who is independent and who can look clearly at the facility and clearly at the family's needs—and most importantly, at the needs of the individual who will be moving into the facility.

"Institutionalization," she says, "creates a kind of dependency and commonality wherein the disabled person does lose much of his individuality. Involving him in decisions and allowing him to take responsibility for his decisions is a process that requires an education and commitment of the facility staff and administration, as well as the understanding of the family. This will take some bold steps on the part of all concerned to ensure that facilities can better serve individual needs."

Suggested reading

Health and Welfare Canada has a series of excellent booklets that explain how to adapt your environment to the special needs of people with various disabilities. Some of the titles: Reaching Aids, Food Preparation Aids, Walking Aids, Bath Lifts, and Dressing Aids. This series of twenty-one booklets is available in English or French.

Also available in English or French is a wonderful book called *Help Yourself! Hints from the Handicapped*, which offers practical advice—and lots of illustrations—on everything from how to buy clothes and cook, to how to play cards if you can't hold the cards.

All are available free of charge from:

Independent Living Series
Communications Directorate
Health and Welfare Canada
Ottawa, Ontario K1A 1B5

LIVING ALONE—AND LIKING IT TOO! [1]
by Mona Winberg, a columnist for the Toronto Sun

"For disabled people, the challenge of living alone has never been as great as it is today.

We are the first generation of persons with disabilities (I have cerebral palsy) to live as long as we do. We share some concerns with the rest of the aging population, but others are uniquely ours.

It is very difficult, for example, to find medical personnel who are knowledgeable about aging among people with a lifelong disability. Doctors are only now beginning to recognize the post-polio syndrome. They are in the dark about other, lesser-known disabilities.

For me, the important quality in choosing a doctor is not how much he knows about handicaps, but rather his attitude. If he has a positive attitude toward you living alone, you will feel much happier and more secure.

It is also extremely important that you make yourself aware of the various support services to which you are entitled. I am a grateful recipient of such vital services as Meals on Wheels and homemaking. They do more than assist me—they enable me to direct my energy and time to tasks that are more essential to me.

Two winters ago I began to have severe pain in my neck and it became necessary to change some of my habits. A physiotherapist suggested that it would help my neck if I didn't go to the library, but asked them to come to me. This has been a tremendous assistance. Not only has my neck been saved the strain of reaching for and carrying books, but I meet some fine people when they deliver them to me.

It was also during this time that I discovered I was entitled to more hours of homemaking help than I was receiving. The services are out there—we just have to make ourselves aware of them.

Another thing that has been helpful is to try and have friends who are supportive and understanding of my desire to live independently. Frankly, I don't have time or patience for people who look on the negative side of everything.

A while ago I read something that has been very meaningful to me. It went like this: Those people are happiest who regard living alone as a privilege, not a punishment.

It's true!"

---

[1] Reprinted with permission from the author.

To sum up . . .

- Disabled people have many of the same needs that the elderly have, and also want to remain independent as long as possible.

- How long a disabled person can remain in his own home depends mainly on the support services available to him—both professional services and those given by family and friends.

- It can sometimes be difficult for disabled people to find the proper care needed to keep them independent, and more is always needed.

- Disabled people who have to move into care facilities can have real problems because the staff doesn't always have the time or the inclination to give them the special care they need. Being the only thirty-year-old among a group of frail eighty-year-olds doesn't help matters.

RESOURCES

If you need help, start with the names on this list. If these people cannot help you, they can tell you where to find the help you need.

Start by requesting the **Senior's Guide to Federal Programs and Services** *and the special guide for your own province. These publications contain a lot of valuable information.*

Seniors' Guide to Federal Programs and Services

Publications Distribution Centre
Health and Welfare Canada
Room 512
Brooke Claxton Building
Tunney's Pasture
Ottawa, Ontario
K1A 0K9
(613) 952-9191

Provincial Seniors' Information Guides

Services Supporting the Independence of Seniors
Contact:

Office for Seniors
Ministry of Health 6-2
1515 Blanshard Street
Victoria, British Columbia
V8W 3C8
(604) 387-2919

Programs for Seniors 1989
Contact:

Seniors Advisory Council
for Alberta 405
Energy Square Building
10109 - 106th Street
Edmonton, Alberta
T5J 3L7
(403) 427-7876

Programs and Services for Seniors— 1988 Directory
Contact:

Saskatchewan Seniors' Secretariat
2151 Scarth Street
Regina, Saskatchewan
S4P 3Z3
(306) 787-5016

Manitoba Senior Citizens' Handbook
Contact:

Manitoba Council on Aging
Manitoba Health
302-333 Broadway Avenue
Winnipeg, Manitoba
R3C 0S9
(204) 945-1997

Guide for Senior Citizens
Contact:

Office for Senior Citizens' Affairs
76 College Street
6th Floor
Toronto, Ontario
M7A 1N3
(416) 965-5106

The Seniors' Guide
Contact:

La Magnetotheque
1030, rue Cherrier
bureau 304
Montreal, Quebec
H2L 1H9
(514) 524-6831

Programs for Seniors
Contact:

Nova Scotia Senior Citizens' Secretariat
P.O. Box 2065
Halifax, Nova Scotia
B3J 2Z1
(902) 424-4649

Resource Manual of Services for
Seniors on Prince Edward Island
Contact:

Division of Aging and Extended Care,
Department of Health and Social
Services
P.O. Box 2000
Charlottetown, P.E.I.
C1A 7N8
(902) 368-4980

Information about Support Services
for Older Adults
Contact:

Division of Services to Senior Citizens
Department of Health
P.O. Box 8700
St. John's, Newfoundland
A1B 4J6
(709) 576-3551

Information Please. . . A Handbook
for Yukon Seniors
Contact:

Department of Health and Human
Resources
Government of Yukon
P.O. Box 2703
Whitehorse, Yukon
Y1A 2C6
(403) 667-5674

Programs and Services for Senior
Citizens
Contact:

Community and Family Support
Service
Northwest Territories Department of
Social Services
Yellowknife, Northwest Territories
X1A 2L9
(403) 873-7707

The Canadian Association of Retired
Persons is a nonprofit national
organization dedicated to improving
the quality of life for Canadians
over 50.
Contact them for membership
information.

Canadian Association of Retired
Persons
27 Queen Street E., Suite 304
Toronto, ON   M5C 2M6
(416) 363-8748

For a free copy of the Canadian
MoneySaver magazine, contact:

Canadian MoneySaver
Box 370
Bath, ON   K0H 1G0
(613) 352-7448

If you have a complicated problem or a serious complaint that cannot be taken care of at the local level, contact these people. They are the ones who are ultimately in charge of issues concerning the care system.

FEDERAL

Consultant Long Term Care
Institutional and Professional Services
Division
Health Services Directorate
Health Services and Promotion Branch
Room 670, Jeanne Mance Building
Tunney's Pasture
Ottawa, Ontario
K1A 1B4
(613) 954-8620

Nursing Consultant
Community Health Services
Health Services and Promotion Branch
Room 606, Jeanne Mance Building
Tunney's Pasture
Ottawa, Ontario
K1A 1B4
(613) 954-8640

Program Analyst
Health Insurance Directorate
Health Services and Promotion Branch
Room 617, Jeanne Mance Building
Tunney's Pasture
Ottawa, Ontario
K1A 1B4
(613) 954-8681

BRITISH COLUMBIA

Executive Director
Office for Seniors
Continuing Care Division
Institutional Services
Ministry of Health
1515 Blanshard Street, 6th Floor
Victoria, British Columbia
V8W 3C8
(604) 387-2286

ALBERTA

Director of Long Term Care Institution
Branch
Alberta Health
Hospital Services Division
Provincial Programs Branch
5th Floor, Hys Centre
11010 - 101 Street
P.O. Box 2222
Edmonton, Alberta
T5J 2P4
(403) 427-7128

Director
Home Care/Community Long Term
Care
Alberta Health
7th Floor, Seventh Street Plaza
10030 - 107th Street
Edmonton, Alberta
T5J 3E4
(403) 427-4610

SASKATCHEWAN

Director, Home Care
Saskatchewan Health
T.C. Douglas Building
3475 Albert Street
Regina, Saskatchewan
S4S 6X6
(306) 787-5010

Executive Director
Continuing Care Branch
Department of Health
3475 Albert Street
Regina, Saskatchewan
S4S 6X6
(306) 787-3629

MANITOBA

Director
Long Term Care Programs Division
Manitoba Health Services Commission
599 Empress Street
Winnipeg, Manitoba
R3C 2T6
(204) 786-7282

Director, Continuing Care Program
Manitoba Health
4th Floor
205-800 Portage Avenue
Winnipeg, Manitoba
R3G 0N4
(204) 945-6736

ONTARIO

Director
Home Services Branch
5th Floor, Hepburn Block
80 Grosvenor Street
Toronto, Ontario
M7A 1E9
(416) 326-9750

Senior Administration Consultant
Institutional Operations Branch
7th Floor
15 Overlea Boulevard
Toronto, Ontario
M4H 1A9
(416) 965-8011

QUEBEC

Chef, Service des programmes a la
communaute
Direction des programmes—
Communaute, famille, jeunesse
Ministere de la Sante et des services
sociaux
1075, chemin Ste-Foy, 6ieme etage
Quebec, Quebec
G1S 2M1
(418) 643-6658

Directeur
Direction des services de longue duree
Ministere de la Sante et des services
sociaux
1075, chemin Ste-Foy, 4ieme etage
Quebec, Quebec
G2S 2M1
(418) 643-6386

NOVA SCOTIA

Administrator
Rehabilitation and Community
Services
Department of Community Services
P.O. Box 696
Halifax, Nova Scotia
B3J 2T7
(902) 424-6762

Assistant Director
Community Health Nursing
Department of Health and Fitness
P.O. Box 488
1690 Hollis Street
Halifax, Nova Scotia
B3J 2R8
(902) 424-4404

NEW BRUNSWICK

Director of Nursing Home Services
Department of Health and Community
Services
P.O. Box 6000
Fredericton, New Brunswick
E3B 5H1
(506) 453-3821

Director
Office for Seniors
Department of Health and Community
Services
P.O. Box 5100
Fredericton, New Brunswick
E3B 5G8
(506) 453-2480

PRINCE EDWARD ISLAND

Director of Home Care and Support
Services
Department of Health and Social
Services
McMillan Building
P.O. Box 2000
Charlottetown, Prince Edward Island
C1A 7N8
(902) 368-4215

NEWFOUNDLAND

Nursing Consultant
Department of Health
Confederation Building
P.O. Box 4750
St. John's, Newfoundland
A1C 5T7
(709) 576-3121

YUKON

Assistant Deputy Minister
Health Services Branch
Health and Human Resources
P.O. Box 2703
Whitehorse, Yukon
Y1A 2C6
(403) 667-5811

Planner (Long Term Care)
Department of Health and Human
Resources
Government of the Yukon
P.O. Box 2703
Whitehorse, Yukon
Y1A 2C6
(403) 667-5857

NORTHWEST TERRITORIES

Head, Policy/Planning
Long-Term Care Rehabilitation
Department of Health
Government of the Northwest
Territories
Yellowknife, Northwest Territories
X1A 2L9
(403) 873-7371

Coordinator Aged and Handicapped
Family and Community Support
Services
Department of Social Services
Government of the Northwest
Territories
Yellowknife, Northwest Territories
X1A 2L9
(403) 873-7707

BRITISH COLUMBIA

BEREAVEMENT SUPPORT

Richmond Golden Age Club
New Horizon Room
Richmond Memorial Community
Centre
Perth Street
Richmond, British Columbia
838-5423
838-2423

CANADIAN ASSOCIATION FOR COMMUNITY LIVING

British Columbians for Mentally
Handicapped People
300 – 30 East 6th Avenue
Vancouver, British Columbia
V5T 4P4
875-1119

CANADIAN MENTAL HEALTH ASSOCIATION

Ms. Pam Simpson
CMHA—100 Mile House Branch
Box 876
100 Mile House, British Columbia
V0K 2E0

Eleanor Shaw
CMHA—Courtney Branch
2716 Virginia Drive
Courtney, British Columbia
V9N 6B3

Ms. Carlene Waugh
CMHA—Cranbrook & District Branch
Box 607
Cranbrook, British Columbia
V1C 4J2

Rene Poirier
CMHA—Trail & District Branch
S.17, C.2, R. R. #1
Fruitvale, British Columbia
V0G 1L0

Mr. Jack Mallow
Administrator
CMHA—Kelowna Branch
Box 535
Kelowna, British Columbia
V1Y 7P1

Mr. Ron Zinck
Administrator
CMHA—Nanaimo Branch
253 Victoria Road
Nanaimo, British Columbia
V9R 2K8

Estelle Pezarro
CMHA—Nelson Branch
604 Fourth Street
Nelson, British Columbia
V1L 2S6

Ms. Frederica Steele
Administrator
CMHA—New Westminster Branch
c/o Bluebird House
408-8th Street
New Westminster, British Columbia
V3M 3R6

Ms. Jo Hannay
Administrator
CMHA—North & West Vancouver
Branch
2132 Hamilton Street
#129
North Vancouver, British Columbia
V7P 2M3

Jean Sherwood
Administrator
CMHA—Penticton Branch
245 Warren Avenue West
Penticton, British Columbia
V2A 7G8

Ms. Marj McConnell
CMHA—Port Alberni Branch
4226-8th Avenue
Port Alberni, British Columbia
V9Y 7S8

Ms. Sue Elliott
CMHA—North Surrey Branch
416 Cardiff Way
Port Moody, British Columbia
V3H 3T1

Ms. Linda Doran
Administrator
CMHA—Prince George Branch
2734 Norwood Street
Prince George, British Columbia
V2L 1Y6

Sany Inness
CMHA—Quesnel
Box 4416
Quesnel, British Columbia
V2J 3J4

Gary Glacken
Executive Director
CMHA—Richmond Branch
6-13680 Bridgeport Road
Richmond, British Columbia
V6V 1V3

Ms. Nancy Parkinson
Administrator
CMHA—Salmon Arm & District Branch
Box 3275
Salmon Arm, British Columbia
V1E 4S1

Ms. Dorothy Braucher
CMHA—Hazelton Branch
Box 9, Braucher Road
South Hazelton, British Columbia
V0J 2R0

Trevoer Thomas
Executive Director
CMHA—Vancouver/Burnaby Branch
1725 West 2nd Avenue
Vancouver, British Columbia
V6J 1H7

Mr. Hugh Bohm
Administrator
CMHA—Vernon & District Branch
3105-28th Avenue
Vernon, British Columbia
V1T 1X8

Gail Simpson
Executive Director
CMHA—Victoria
1450 Elford Street
Victoria, British Columbia
V8S 3S8

Cindy Barrett
Administrator
CMHA—White Rock/South Surrey
Branch
1159 Vidal Street
White Rock, British Columbia
V4B 3T4

Gail Gustafson
Administrator
CMHA—Williams Lake
305-197 Second Avenue North
Williams Lake, British Columbia
V2G 1Z7

FAMILY SERVICE CANADA

Catholic Community Services
150 Robson Street
Vancouver, British Columbia
V6B 2A7
683-0281

North Shore Family Services Society
303-126 East 15th Street
North Vancouver, British Columbia
V7L 2P9
988-5281

Pacific Centre for Human Development
3221 Heatherbell Road
Victoria, British Columbia
V9C 1Y8
478-8357

MEALS ON WHEELS

*If your city is listed here, there is a
Meals on Wheels program there. If
there's no phone number listed, just
look in your local telephone directory
or ask any health professional in your
area.*

Abbotsford

Agassiz

Armstrong, 546-3465

Brentwood Bay

Burnaby

Campbell River

Castlegar, 365-2148

Chemainus

Chilliwack

Comox

Cranbrook, 489-4751
Creston, 428-2113
Dawson Creek
Delta
Duncan
Fernie, 423-6910
Fort St. John
Ganges
Golden, 344-5462
Grand Forks, 442-5544
Hope
Kelowna, 762-9989
Keremeos, 499-5679
Kimberley, 427-2317
Ladysmith
Lake Cowichan
Langley
Maple Ridge
Merritt
Mission
Nakusp, 265-3674
Nanaimo
Naramata
Nelson, 352-2911
New Denver, 358-7711
New Westminster
Okanagan Falls
Oliver
Osoyoos
Parksville
Penticton
Port Alberni
Powell River
Prince George
Prince Rupert
Princeton
Victorian Order of Nurses
RichmondVancouver Branch
Rossland, 362-5530
Salmon Arm, 832-2182
Sechelt
Sidney
Sooke
Sparwood, 425-6387

Summerland
Surrey
Terrace
Trail, 362-5530
Little Mountain Neighbourhood
House Society, Vancouver
Vernon, 545-9288
James Bay Community School Society
Victoria
Silver Threads Service, Victoria
West Vancouver
White Rock

OCCUPATIONAL THERAPISTS

B.C. Society of Occupational
Therapists (BCSOT)
Suite 222
4585 Canada Way
Burnaby, British Columbia
V5G 4L6
294-2717

RED CROSS

Canadian Red Cross Society
B.C.–Yukon
4710 Kingsway
Suite 400
Burnaby, British Columbia
V5H 4M2

SELF-HELP CLEARING HOUSES

Self Help Collaboration Project
1625 W. 8th Avenue
Vancouver, British Columbia
V6J 1T9
731-7781

SELF-HELP GROUPS

Aids Vancouver
1272 Richards Street
Vancouver, British Columbia
V6B 3G2
687-5220

Alzheimer Society of B.C.
20-601 W. Cordova Street
Vancouver, British Columbia
V6B 1G1
681-6530

Alzheimer Support Group
Margaret Fultron Centre
1044 St. Georges Street
North Vancouver, British Columbia
V7L 3H6
929-4244

American Association of Marriage &
Family Therapists
2454 West 13th Avenue
Vancouver, British Columbia
V6K 2S8
731-2952

Arthritis Society
North Shore Branch
308-2020 Belview
North Vancouver, British Columbia
V7N 4E5
925-1148

Brain Tumor Support Group
Cancer Control Agency of B.C.
600 W. 10th Avenue
Vancouver, British Columbia
V5Z 4E6
877-6000

British Columbia and Yukon
Heart Foundation
1212 West Broadway
Vancouver, British Columbia
V6H 3V2
736-4404

Can-Cope
Chronic Pain and Disability Society
Vancouver, British Columbia
263-8798

Cansurmount
Canadian Cancer Society
565 W. 10th Avenue
Vancouver, British Columbia
V5Z 4J4
872-4400

Caregiver's Support Group
Mount St. Joseph's Hospital
3080 Prince Edward Street
Vancouver, British Columbia
V5T 3N4

BC Coalition of Disabled
211-456 W. Broadway
Vancouver, British Columbia
V5Y 1R3
875-0188

Elder's Network
105-2182 W. 12th Avenue
Vancouver, British Columbia
V6K 2N4
733-4169

Family Support Institute
300-30 E. 6th Avenue
Vancouver, British Columbia
V5T 4P4
875-1119

Information Services Vancouver
202-3102 Main Street
Vancouver, British Columbia
V5T 3G7
(875-6381)

Life Resource Centre
101-395 W. Broadway
Vancouver, British Columbia
V5Y 1A7
873-5013

Living With Cancer
Cancer Control Agency of B.C.
600 W.10th Avenue
Vancouver, British Columbia
V5Z 4E6
877-6000 #2194

Living With Cancer
Vancouver, British Columbia
581-5701

Mature Women's Network
2nd Floor
411 Dunsmuir Street
Vancouver, British Columbia
V6B 1X4
681-3986

The Multiple Sclerosis Society
of Canada
British Columbia Division 18
December 1990
Suite 205
6125 Sussex Avenue
Burnaby, British Columbia
V5H 4G1
437-3244

Multiple Sclerosis Support Group
Highlands United Church
3255 Edgemont Blvd.
North Vancouver, British Columbia
984-6318

Multiple Sclerosis Support Group
(Surrey)
Newton Royal Canadian Legion
13564-73 Avenue
Surrey, British Columbia

Ostop Society of British Columbia
203-2182 W. 12th Avenue
Vancouver, British Columbia
V6K 2N4
731-4997

BC Parkinson's Disease Association
Vancouver Neurological Centre
1195 W. 8th Avenue
Vancouver, British Columbia
V6H 1C5
734-2221

Richmond Volunteer Centre
Suite 100
4040 #3 Road
Richmond, British Columbia
V6X 2C2

Vancouver Persons with Aids Coalition
P.O. Box 136
1215 Davie Street
Vancouver, British Columbia
V6E 1N4
683-3381

The Vancouver Volunteer Centre
Suite 301
3102 Main Street
Vancouver, British Columbia
V5T 3G7
875-9144

Victoria Volunteer Bureau
211-620 View Street
Victoria, British Columbia
V8W 1J6
386-2269

West End Multiple Sclerosis
Self-Help Group
501-1515 Granville Street
Vancouver, British Columbia
V6Z 2M8

West End Seniors' Network
Barclay Manor
1447 Barclay
Vancouver, British Columbia
V6G 1J6
669-7339

White Rock Parkinson's
Self Help Group
White Rock Senior Citizens'
Activity Centre
1475 Kent Street
White Rock, British Columbia
V4B 3W5
538-1912

WHO (Widows Helping Others)
Dogwood Pavilion
624 Poirier Street
Coquitlam, British Columbia
V3J 6A9
936-1737

Widows' Network
c/o 102-250 18th Street
West Vancouver, British Columbia
V7V 3V5
925-1513

ALBERTA

CANADIAN ASSOCIATION FOR COMMUNITY LIVING

Alberta Association for
Community Living
11728 Kingsway Avenue
Edmonton, Alberta
T5G 0X5
451-3055

CANADIAN MENTAL HEALTH ASSOCIATION

Ms. Martha Winchell
Staff Contact
CMHA—Barrhead Branch
c/o F.C.S.S.
Box 488
5115-45 Street
Barrhead, Alberta
T0G 0E0

Ms. Trish Turnball
Regional Director
Alberta Central Region
5015-48 Street North West
#2
Calgary, Alberta
T2N 2A4

Ms. Trish Cameron
Regional Director
Alberta South Central Region
723-14 Street North West
#201
Calgary, Alberta
T2N 2A4

Ms. Betty Frieson
Staff Contact
CMHA—Claresholm Branch
Box 1354
Claresholm, Alberta
T0L 0T0

Mr. Brian Bechtel
Regional Director
Alberta North Central Region
10010-112 Street
9th Floor
Edmonton, Alberta
T5K 2J1

Simonne Walsh
Staff Contact
CMHA—Fort McMurray Branch
c/o Peter Pond Community School
Room 22B
9601 Franklin Avenue
Fort McMurray, Alberta
T9H 2J8

Tina Rogers
Regional Director
Alberta North Region
10118-101 Avenue
#201
Grande Prairie, Alberta
T8V 0Y2

Ms. Val Boehme
Regional Director
Alberta South Region
505-7th Street South
Lethbridge, Alberta
T1J 2G8

Staff Contact
CMHA—Lloydminster Branch
5211-50th Street
Lloydminster, Alberta
T9V 0M4

Mr. Darren Rud
Regional Director
Alberta South East Region
379 Aberdeen Street South East
Medicine Hat, Alberta
T1A 0R3

Ms. A. Bloomquist
CMHA—Brooks Branch
General Delivery
Scandia, Alberta
T0J 2Z0

FAMILY AND COMMUNITY SUPPORT SERVICES

Airdrie, 948-5907
Alix, 747-2030
Assumption, 321-3767
Athabasca, 675-2623
Banff, 762-4426
Barrhead, 674-3341
Bassano, 641-3520
Beaumont, 929-8782
Beaverlodge, 354-2938
Berwyn, 338-3801
Black Diamond, 933-4340
Blairmore, 362-8862
Bon Accord, 921-3550
Bonnyville, 826-2120
826-3333
Bow Island, 545-2656
Breton, 696-3636
Brocket, 965-3802
Brooks, 362-3333
Bruderheim, 796-3731
Calgary, 265-0661
266-6200
268-5111
Camrose, 672-7022
672-0141
Canmore, 678-5597
Caroline, 722-2341
Carstairs, 337-3341
Caslan, 689-2170
Castor, 882-2115
Claresholm, 625-4417
Coaldale, 327-6507
Cochrane, 932-2075
Cold Lake, 639-3626
Coleman, 562-8862
Coronation, 578-3022
Crossfield, 946-5565
Didsbury, 335-3311
Drayton Valley, 542-7777
Drumheller, 823-6300
Dunmore, 526-2888
Eckville, 746-3177

Edmonton, 423-5510
428-5917
Edson, 723-4401
Elk Point, 724-3800
Fairview, 835-5461
Falher, 837-8311
Foremost, 867-3733
Fort Assiniboine, 584-3922
Fort Chipewyan, 697-3674
Fort Macleod, 553-4401
Fort McMurray, 743-7921
Fort Saskatchewan, 998-2266
Fort Vermilion, 927-4340
Fox Creek, 622-3896
Frog Lake, 943-2211
Gibbons, 923-3331
Gleichen, 734-3040
Glendon, 635-3807
Glenevis, 967-2225
Goodfish Lake, 636-3622
Grand Centre, 594-5024
594-1471
Grande Cache, 827-2296
Grande Prairie, 539-6255
532-9722
538-0409
Granum, 687-3822
Hanna, 854-4700
High Level, 926-2267
High Prairie, 523-4401
523-4441
High River, 652-2110
Hinton, 865-2217
Hobbema, 585-3793
Hythe, 356-3888
Innisfail, 227-3376
Irricana, 935-4672
Jasper, 852-5386
Jean D'Or, 759-3912
Killam, 385-3976
La Crete, 928-3967
Lac La Biche, 623-2130
Lacombe, 782-6637
Leduc, 986-2251
986-2261

Lethbridge, 320-2222
320-3020
Lloydminster, 875-9127
Ma-Me-O Beach, 586-2251
Mannville, 763-3005
Medicine Hat, 529-8383
529-8311
Medley, 594-6006
Millet, 387-5111
Mirror, 788-2415
Morinville, 939-5887
939-4321
939-4361
Morley, 881-3770
Nampa, 322-3954
Nanton, 646-2436
Okotoks, 938-4404
Olds, 556-6981
Onoway, 967-5338
Paddle Prairie, 981-2342
Peace River, 624-1000
Pincher Creek, 627-2232
Ponoka, 783-4462
Provost, 753-2280
Rainbow Lake, 956-3880
Raymond, 752-3303
Red Deer, 343-6074
342-8100
Redcliff, 548-3618
Rimbey, 843-2030
Rocky Mountain House, 845-3720
989-3943
989-3740
Saddle Lake, 726-3829
Sexsmith, 568-4345
Sherwood Park, 464-4044
Slave Lake, 849-5325
Smoky Lake, 656-2255
Spruce Grove, 962-2611
Sputinow, 943-2575
St. Albert, 458-2771
459-1505
St. Paul, 645-5311
Standard, 644-3839
Standoff, 737-3974

Stavely, 549-3761
Stettler, 742-2337
Stony Plain, 963-9770
Strathmore, 934-5335
Sundre, 638-3220
Swan Hills, 333-4304
Sylvan Lake, 887-2141
Taber, 223-4403
Thorhild, 398-3688
Three Hills, 443-5454
Tilley, 377-2203
Tofield, 662-3269
Turner Valley, 933-4945
Two Hills, 657-3540
Valleyview, 524-3924
Vegreville, 632-3966
Vermilion, 853-2091
Viking, 336-4024
Vulcan, 485-2192
Wainwright, 842-2777
842-2555
Warner, 642-3737
Westlock, 349-5900
Wetaskiwin, 352-6023
352-3321
Whitecourt, 778-6300
Wildwood, 325-3782
Winterburn, 470-5666
Zama, 683-2237

FAMILY SERVICE CANADA

Calgary Family Service Bureau
120-13th Avenue South East
Calgary, Alberta
T2G 1B3
233-2370

Catholic Social Services
8815-99th Street
Edmonton, Alberta
T6E 3V3
432-1137

Family Service Association
of Edmonton
9912-106 Street
Edmonton, Alberta
T5K 1E2
423-2831

Lethbridge Family Services
3rd Floor
515-7th Street South
Lethbridge, Alberta
T1J 2G8
327-5724

Red Deer Family Service Bureau
304-5000 Gaetz Avenue
Red Deer, Alberta
T4N 6C2
343-6400

MEALS ON WHEELS

*If your city is listed here, there is a
Meals on Wheels program there. If
there's no phone number listed, just
look in your local telephone directory
or ask any health professional in your
area.*

Athabasca, Alberta

Banff, Alberta

Barrhead, Alberta

Beaumont, Alberta

Beaverlodge, Alberta

Bonneville, Alberta

Bowden, Alberta

Calgary, Alberta

Camrose, Alberta

Cold Lake, Alberta

Devon, Alberta

Didsbury, Alberta

Drayton Valley, Alberta

Drumheller, Alberta

Eckville, Alberta

Edson, Alberta

Elk Point, Alberta

Fort Saskatchewan, Alberta

Gibbons, Alberta

Glendon, Alberta

Grand Prairie, Alberta

High Level, Alberta

High River, Alberta

Hinton, Alberta

Innisfail, Alberta

Jasper, Alberta

Killam, Alberta

La Crete, Alberta

Barbara Jeffery

Lacombe, Alberta

Lamont, Alberta

Leduc, Alberta

Lethbridge, Alberta

Mannville, Alberta

Medicine Hat, Alberta

Peace River, Alberta

Provost, Alberta

Red Deer, Alberta

Redwater, Alberta

Rimby, Alberta

Saddle Lake, Alberta

Sherwood Park, Alberta

Slave Lake, Alberta

Spruce Grove, Alberta

St. Albert, Alberta

St. Paul, Alberta

Stettler, Alberta

Stony Plain, Alberta

Two Hills, Alberta

Vegreville, Alberta

Viking, Alberta

Wainwright, Alberta

OCCUPATIONAL THERAPISTS

Alberta Association of Registered
Occupational Therapists (AAROT)
Suite 300, Centre 104
5241 Calgary Trail
Edmonton, Alberta
T6H 5G8
436-8381

RED CROSS

Canadian Red Cross Society
Alberta-Northwest Territories
737-13th Avenue Southwest
Calgary, Alberta
T2R 1J1

SELF-HELP

Alberta Council on Aging
Room 501, Liberty Building
10506 Jasper Avenue
Edmonton, Alberta
T5J 2W9
423-7781

Alberta Pensioners and Senior
Citizens Organization
c/o Secretary-Treasurer
Irene Newman
Box 1411
Claresholm, Alberta
T0L 0T0
625-3175

CNIB Calgary Service Centre
15 Colonel Baker Place NE
Calgary, Alberta
T2E 4Z3
488-4871

CNIB Lethbridge Service Centre
206, 542-7 Street South
Lethbridge, Alberta
T1J 2H1
327-1044

Canadian Pensioners
Concerned, Alberta Division
907, 4440-106 Street
Edmonton, Alberta
T6H 4X1
(436-7837)

Family and Community
Support Services Branch
Family and Social Services
6th Floor, Donsdale Place
10709 Jasper Avenue
Edmonton, Alberta
T5J 3N3
427-2803

Home Adaptation Program
Housing Division
Alberta Municipal Affairs
P.O. Box 3120
Edmonton, Alberta
T5J 4L8
427-8161

Mental Health Office
Calgary Region
206 Hillhurst Professional Building
301-14 Street, N.W.
Calgary, Alberta
T2N 2A4

Mental Health Office
South Region
2105-20 Avenue
P.O. Box 60
Coaldale, Alberta
T0K 0L0
381-5329

Mental Health Office
Edmonton Region
5th Floor, 108 Street Building
9942-108 Street
Edmonton, Alberta
T5K 2J5
427-4444

Mental Health Office
Northeast Region
9th Floor, Provincial Building
9915 Franklin Avenue
Fort McMurray, Alberta
T9H 2K4
743-7450

Mental Health Office
Northwest Region
6th Floor, Nordic Court
10014-99 Street
Grande Prairie, Alberta
T8V 3N4
538-5160

Mental Health Office
Central Region
2nd Floor, 4920-51 Street
Red Deer, Alberta
T4N 6K8
340-5047

Senior District Medical Officer
Veterans Affairs Canada
Sam Livingston Building
Main Floor
510-12 Avenue S.W.
Calgary, Alberta
T2R 0X5
292-4048

Senior District Medical Officer
Veterans Affairs Canada
940 Canada Place
9700 Jasper Avenue
Edmonton, Alberta
T5J 4C3
495-3762

Seniors' Emergency Medical
Alert Program
Housing Division
Alberta Municipal Affairs
P.O. Box 3040
Edmonton, Alberta
T5J 4L7
422-1809

Victorian Order of Nurses
417-14 Street
Calgary, Alberta
T2N 2A1
283-2819

Victorian Order of Nurses
7211-96A Avenue
Edmonton, Alberta
T6B 1B5
466-0293

Victorian Order of Nurses
419, 909-3 Avenue N.
Lethbridge, Alberta
T1H 0H5
328-0033

Victorian Order of Nurses
666-5th Street S.W.
Medicine Hat, Alberta
T1A 4H6
529-8025

SELF-HELP CLEARING HOUSES

Family Life Education Council
233-12th Avenue S.W.
Calgary, Alberta
T2R 0G9
262-1117

SELF-HELP GROUPS

Acadia Aquatic Seniors Club
10004-5 Street S.E.
Calgary, Alberta
271-2196

Advice, Information and
Direction Centre
Box 2100
Calgary, Alberta
T2P 2M5
265-3411

After Hours Social Services
Alberta Social Services
2nd Floor
811-14 Street N.W.
Calgary, Alberta
270-5333

Aid Service of Edmonton
203, 10711-107 Avenue
Edmonton, Alberta
426-3242

Alberta Mortgage and Housing
Corporation
2924-11 Street N.E.
Calgary, Alberta
250-4600

Alzheimer Association of Alberta
Suite 612
1701 Centre Street N.W.
Calgary, Alberta
T2E 7Y2
277-1501

American Association of Marriage &
Family Therapists
P.O. Box s4853
Edmonton, Alberta
T6E 5G7
963-6151

Banff Trail Community Seniors
2115-20 Avenue N.W.
Calgary, Alberta
289-4963

Bow Cliff Seniors
608 Poplar Road S.W.
Calgary, Alberta
286-4488

Bowmont Seniors' Assistance
Association
5000 Bowness Road N.W.
Calgary, Alberta
268-1811

Bridgeland We-Care Centre
736 McDougall Court N.E.
Calgary, Alberta
264-5512

Calgary Chinese Elderly
Citizens Association
Basement
102-3 Avenue S.W.
Calgary, Alberta
268-6122

Calgary Community Support Services
for Seniors
807-6 Street S.E.
Calgary, Alberta
262-3388

Calgary Fun Finders Pioneers Club
919 McDougall Road N.E.
Calgary, Alberta
264-1269

Calgary Home Care Program
Calgary, Alberta
228-7480

Calgary Housing Authority
1701 Centre Street N.W.
Calgary, Alberta
221-9100

Calgary Jewish Centre
1607-90 Avenue S.W.
Calgary, Alberta
253-8600

Calgary Meals on Wheels
3610 Macleod Trail S.E.
Calgary, Alberta
243-2834

Calgary Parks & Recreation
Centre West Area Office
Calgary, Alberta
248-4331

Calgary Parks & Recreation
East Area Office
Calgary, Alberta
272-3301

Calgary Parks & Recreation
North Area Office
Calgary, Alberta
289-8418

Calgary Parks & Recreation
Senior Citizens' Transportation
Services
Calgary, Alberta
268-1385

Calgary Parks & Recreation
Seniors Section
Calgary, Alberta
268-5213

Calgary Parks & Recreation
South Area Office
Calgary, Alberta
253-4752

Calgary Recreation & Culture
Association for Seniors (CRCA)
722-16 Avenue N.E.
Calgary, Alberta
230-1801

Calhome Properties
12th Floor
800 Macleod Trail S.E.
Calgary, Alberta
268-1450

Care West
1070 McDougall Road N.E.
Calgary, Alberta
267-2900

City Centre Seniors
720-1 Street S.W.
Calgary, Alberta
269-1223

Community Health Nursing Services
Calgary, Alberta
228-7550

Community Social Workers
Albert Park/Radisson Heights
Calgary, Alberta
273-4141

Community Social Workers
Bowness
Calgary, Alberta
288-7701

Community Social Workers
Connaught
Calgary, Alberta
244-4267

Community Social Workers
Downtown Outreach
Calgary, Alberta
268-5175

Community Social Workers
Forest Lawn
Calgary, Alberta
273-4141

Community Social Workers
Heritage Square
Calgary, Alberta
253-7456

Community Social Workers
Inglewood
Calgary, Alberta
264-2484

Community Social Workers
Shaganappi
Calgary, Alberta
268-5165

Community Social Workers
Thornhill
Calgary, Alberta
274-8543

Community Social Workers
Village Square
Calgary, Alberta
293-1557

Confederation Park Senior
Citizens Centre
2212-13 Street N.W.
Calgary, Alberta
289-4780

Crossroads 50 + Club
1803-14 Avenue N.E.
Calgary, Alberta
277-9089

Family and Community Support
Services
City of Calgary Social Services
Department
Calgary, Alberta
268-5111

Fifty-five + Club
Brentwood Community
5107-33 Street N.W.
Calgary, Alberta
284-3477

Filipino Calgarian Seniors Club
Calgary, Alberta
252-9018

Fish Creek Seniors
8038 Fairmount Drive S.E.
Calgary, Alberta
253-4744

Forest Lawn Seniors Outreach
3810-17 Avenue S.E.
Calgary, Alberta
273-4141

The Friendship Circle
12, 240-15 Avenue S.W.
Calgary, Alberta
265-0204

Glamorgan 55 Plus Seniors Club
4207-46 Avenue S.W.
Calgary, Alberta
242-5766

Glowing Embers Club
313-3600 Sarcee Road S.W.
Calgary, Alberta
240-2175

Golden Age Club
610-8 Avenue S.E.
Calgary, Alberta
262-6342

Golden Friendship
4335-69 Street N.W.
Calgary, Alberta
288-6991

The Good Companions
2609-19 Avenue S.W.
Calgary, Alberta
249-6991

Greater Forest Lawn Senior
Citizens Society
3425-26 Avenue S.E.
Calgary, Alberta
272-4661

Guys and Dolls
4740-17 Avenue N.W.
Calgary, Alberta
288-3131

Haysboro Fifty Plus Club
1204-89 Avenue S.W.
Calgary, Alberta
253-1563

Healthcare & Rehab Specialties
Bridgeland Corner
#1, 630-1st Avenue N.E.
Calgary, Alberta
262-7595; 1-800-232-9408

Healthcare & Rehab Specialties
Kingsway Professional Centre
114, 10611 Kingsway
Edmonton, Alberta
T5G 3C8
424-6094; 1-800-232-9408

Heart and Stroke Foundation of Alberta
1825 Park Road S.E.
Calgary, Alberta
T2G 3Y6
264-5549

Highwood Seniors
Harlow Avenue and Hudson Road N.W.
Calgary, Alberta
289-9329 or 289-0317

Hillhurst/Sunnyside Seniors Social
and Recreation Club
1118 Kensington Road N.W.
Calgary, Alberta
283-0554

Homemaker Service
Calgary Family Service Bureau
#200, 707-10 Avenue S.W.
Calgary, Alberta
269-9888

Huntington Pioneers Association
520-78 Avenue N.W.
Calgary, Alberta
275-4294

Information Centre
City of Calgary Social Services
Department
Calgary, Alberta
268-4656

Inglewood Silver Threads Association
1311-9 Avenue S.W.
Calgary, Alberta
264-1006

Kerby Centre
1133-7 Avenue S.W.
Calgary, Alberta
265-0661

Know Your Neighbour Club
924 Heritage Drive S.W.
Calgary, Alberta
259-4080

Metropolitan Calgary Foundation
110-10 Avenue N.W.
Calgary, Alberta
276-5541

The Multiple Sclerosis Society of
Canada
Alberta Division
2nd Floor
11203 70th Street
Edmonton, Alberta
T5B 1T1
471-3313

Neighbourhood Help
Hillhurst/Sunnyside Community
Association
1118 Kensington Road N.W.
Calgary, Alberta
283-0554

Nutrition Consultation
Calgary, Alberta
228-7420

Ogden House Senior Citizens' Club
7609-20A Street S.E.
Calgary, Alberta
279-2003

Open Door Senior Fellowship
513-13 Avenue S.W.
Calgary, Alberta
269-7900

Outreach Project for Eastern Core
Seniors (OPECS)
602-1 Street S.E.
Calgary, Alberta
269-3183 or 269-2212

Outreach Services
Calgary Public Library
616 Macleod Trail S.E.
Calgary, Alberta
260-2702; TDD 264-8021

Parkdale Nifty Fifties Social Club
3512-5 Avenue N.W.
Calgary, Alberta
283-0620

Parkridge Sundowners
222 Burroughs Circle N.E.
Calgary, Alberta
293-4557

Project Home Help
City of Calgary Social Services
Department
311-34 Avenue S.E.
Calgary, Alberta
243-2757

Public Health Inspection
Calgary, Alberta
228-7570

Ramsay Welcome Centre
1140-8 Street S.E.
Calgary, Alberta
263-2277

Renfrew Sixty Plus Club
1318 Regal Crescent N.E.
Calgary, Alberta
276-4747

Senior Citizens' Central Council
922-9 Avenue S.E.
Calgary, Alberta
266-6200

Senior Liaison Program
Calgary Police Service
6th Floor
133-6th Avenue S.E.
Calgary, Alberta
268-8398

Seniors Assisting Seniors (SAS)
Confederation Park
2212-13 Street N.W.
Calgary, Alberta
289-4780

Shalem Manor
3010-51 Street S.W.
Calgary, Alberta
246-5519

Shopping Services for
the Frail and Elderly
City of Calgary Social Services
Department
311-34 Avenue S.E.
Calgary, Alberta
243-0850

South Calgary Community Seniors
3130-16 Street S.W.
Calgary, Alberta
244-5411

Southwood Seniors (55 Plus) Club
11 Sackville Drive S.W.
Calgary, Alberta
253-4846

Special Needs Taxi Service
Social Services Department
City of Calgary
Calgary, Alberta
268-5176

St. Andrews "In-Group"
2504-13 Avenue N.W.
Calgary, Alberta
282-5211

St. Mary's Seniors
219-18 Avenue S.W.
Calgary, Alberta
228-4170

Thornview Seniors
5600 Centre Street North
Calgary, Alberta
275-0300

Triwood Tri-Liters
2244 Chicoutimi Drive N.W.
Calgary, Alberta
282-2677

Upper Valley Seniors
1602, 135 Lynnview Road S.E.
Calgary, Alberta
279-0056

Varsity Seniors Club
4103 Varsity Drive N.W.
Calgary, Alberta
288-9001

Victorian Order of Nurses
110C, 1330-15 Avenue S.W.
Calgary, Alberta
245-3050

Village Square Seniors' Society
2623-56 Street N.E.
Calgary, Alberta
285-3364

The Volunteer Action Centre
9844-110 Street
Edmonton, Alberta
T5K 1J2
482-6431

Volunteer Centre of Calgary
Suite 201
110-11th Street South East
Calgary, Alberta
T2G 0X5
265-5633

West Hillhurst Go-Getters Assoc.
1940-6 Avenue N.W.
Calgary, Alberta
283-3720

West Mount Pleasant 50 & Over Club
602-22 Avenue N.W.
Calgary, Alberta
289-5085

Westside Seniors' Service Centre
134 Scarboro Avenue S.W.
Calgary, Alberta
244-1100

Widowed Services
Calgary Family Service Bureau
#310, 707-10 Avenue S.W.
Calgary, Alberta
233-2370

Wild Rose Seniors
4411-10 Avenue S.W.
Calgary, Alberta
242-0212

Work Activity Project
City of Calgary Social Services
Department
311-34 Avenue S.E.
Calgary, Alberta
243-1501

SASKATCHEWAN

ADULT DAY CARE PROGRAMS

Centennial Special Care Home
Langenburg, Saskatchewan
734-2232

Foyer D'Youville Home
Gravelbourg, Saskatchewan
648-3185

Humboldt and District
Housing Corporation
Humboldt, Saskatchewan
682-2628

Lutheran Sunset Home
Saskatoon, Saskatchewan
652-8566

Nipawin District Nursing Home Inc.
Nipawin, Saskatchewan
862-9828

Northern Housing Development
(1973) Inc.
Prince Albert, Saskatchewan
764-7777

Oliver Lodge
Saskatoon, Saskatchewan
382-4111

Parkridge Centre
Saskatoon, Saskatchewan
978-2333

Regina Pioneer Village Ltd.
Regina, Saskatchewan
757-5646

The Salvation Army
Regina, Saskatchewan
543-0655

Sherbrooke Community Centre
Saskatoon, Saskatchewan
374-7955

St. Anthony's Home
Moose Jaw, Saskatchewan
692-7874

Wawota & District Special
Care Home Inc.
Wawota, Saskatchewan
739-2400

CANADIAN ASSOCIATION FOR COMMUNITY LIVING
Saskatchewan Association for the
Mentally Retarded
3031 Louise Street
Saskatoon Saskatchewan
S7J 3L1
955-3344

CANADIAN MENTAL HEALTH ASSOCIATION
Staff Contact
CMHA—Duck Lake Branch
Box 370
Duck Lake, Saskatchewan
S0K 1J0

Staff Contact
CMHA—Estevan Branch
1034-1st Street
Estevan, Saskatchewan
S4A 0G8

Ms. Mary Ann Poletz
Staff Contact
CMHA—Kindersley Branch
Box 244
101-105 5th Avenue East
Kindersley, Saskatchewan
S0L 1S0

Ms. Peggy Johnson
Staff Contact
CMHA—Moose Jaw Branch
30 Caribou Street West
Moose Jaw, Saskatchewan
S6H 2J6

Ms. Gayle Nicholaichuk
Staff Contact
CMHA—Battleford Branch
1342-100th Street
North Battleford, Saskatchewan
S9A 0V8

Ms. Gloria Mitchell
Staff Contact
CMHA—Prince Albert Branch
40 11th Street East
Prince Albert, Saskatchewan
S6V 0Z9

Mr. Ian Andrew
Staff Contact
CMHA—Saskatoon Branch
310 Idywyld Drive North
Room 210
Saskatoon, Saskatchewan
S7L 0Z2

Staff Contact
CMHA—Shellbrook Branch
Stump Lake, Saskatchewan
S0J 2S0

Ms. Donna Schultz-Abel
Staff Contact
CMHA—Swift Current Branch
391 2nd Avenue N.W.
Swift Current, Saskatchewan
S9H 0P5

Ms. Shirley Kerr
Staff Contact
CMHA—Weyburn Branch
404 Ashford Street
Weyburn, Saskatchewan
S4H 1K1

Ms. Lorna Boyce
Staff Contact
CMHA—Yorkton Branch
Box 997
Yorkton, Saskatchewan
S3N 2X3

FAMILY SERVICE CANADA

Catholic Family Service Society
of Regina
395-15th Avenue
Regina, Saskatchewan
S4N 0V1
525-0521

Catholic Family Services of Saskatoon
500-333 3rd Avenue North
Saskatoon, Saskatchewan
S7K 2H9
244-7773

Family Service Bureau of Regina
1801 Toronto Street
Regina, Saskatchewan
S4P 1M7
757-6675

Saskatoon Family Service Bureau
450-350 3rd Avenue North
Saskatoon, Saskatchewan
S7K 1M4
244-0127

HOME CARE

Biggar, 948-3379
Broadview, 696-2500
Canora, 563-5656
Canwood, 468-2290
Carlyle, 453-6740
Carnduff, 482-5105
Esterhazy, 745-6700
Estevan, 634-7337
Foam Lake, 272-3338
Fort San, 332-6683
Gravelbourg, 648-2234
Humboldt, 682-2609
Indian Head, 695-2244
Kindersley, 463-4944
Kyle, 375-2400
Lanigan, 365-3400
Leader, 628-3398
Lestock, 274-2034
Lloydminster, 825-7070
Luseland, 372-4313
Maple Creek, 662-3600
Marcelin, 226-2028

Meadow Lake, 236-6600
Melfort, 752-9511
Melville, 728-5125
Moose Jaw, 694-0612
Moosomin, 435-3888
Nipawin, 862-9822
North Battleford, 445-3795
Outlook, 867-9633
Pelly, 595-2092
Prince Albert, 933-2969
Quill Lake, 383-4124
Regina, 586-0355
Rosetown, 882-4175
Saskatoon, 934-2112
Shaunavon, 397-2648
Swift Current, 773-3161
Tisdale, 873-5950
Unity, 228-3788
Wakaw, 233-5292
Watrous, 946-3921
Weyburn, 842-6870
Willow Bunch, 473-2221
Yorkton, 782-3003

MEALS ON WHEELS

*If your city is listed here, there is a
Meals on Wheels program there. If
there's no phone number listed, just
look in your local telephone directory
or ask any health professional in your
area.*

Biggar, Saskatchewan
Broadview, Saskatchewan
Canora, Saskatchewan
Canwood, Saskatchewan
Carlyle, Saskatchewan
Carnduff, Saskatchewan
Esterhazy, Saskatchewan
Estevan, Saskatchewan
Foam Lake, Saskatchewan
Fort Qu'Appelle, Saskatchewan
Gravelbourg, Saskatchewan
Humboldt, Saskatchewan
Indian Head, Saskatchewan

Kindersley, Saskatchewan
Kyle, Saskatchewan
Lanigan, Saskatchewan
Leader, Saskatchewan
Lestock, Saskatchewan
Lloydminster, Saskatchewan
Luseland, Saskatchewan
Maple Creek, Saskatchewan
Marcelin, Saskatchewan
Meadow Lake, Saskatchewan
Melfort, Saskatchewan
Melville, Saskatchewan
Moose Jaw, Saskatchewan
Moosomin, Saskatchewan
Nipawin, Saskatchewan
North Battleford, Saskatchewan
Outlook, Saskatchewan
Pelly, Saskatchewan
Prince Albert, Saskatchewan
Quill Lake, Saskatchewan
Regina, Saskatchewan
Rosetown, Saskatchewan
Saskatoon, Saskatchewan
Shaunavon, Saskatchewan
Swift Current, Saskatchewan
Tisdale, Saskatchewan
Unity, Saskatchewan
Wakaw, Saskatchewan
Watrous, Saskatchewan
Weyburn, Saskatchewan
Willow Bunch, Saskatchewan
Yorkton, Saskatchewan

OCCUPATIONAL THERAPISTS

Saskatchewan Society of Occupational
Therapists (SSOT)
c/o Plains Health Centre
4500 Wascana Parkway
Regina, Saskatchewan
S4S 5W9
584-6304

RED CROSS

Canadian Red Cross Society
Saskatchewan
2571 Broad Street
P.O. Box 1185
Regina, Saskatchewan
S4P 3B4

SELF-HELP CLEARING HOUSES

Self Help Development Unit
410 Cumberland Avenue North
Saskatoon, Saskatchewan
S7M 1M6
652-7817

SELF-HELP GROUPS

Alzheimer Association of
Saskatchewan
238-408 Broad Street
Regina, Saskatchewan
S4R 1X3
949-4141

Continuing Care
122-3rd Avenue North
Saskatoon, Saskatchewan
S7K 2H6

Heart and Stroke Foundation of
Saskatchewan
279-3rd Avenue North
Saskatoon, Saskatchewan
S7K 2H8
244-2124

The Multiple Sclerosis Society
of Canada
Saskatchewan Division
2329 11th Avenue
Regina, Saskatchewan
S4P 0K2
522-5607

Volunteer Bureau of Regina
2231 Broad Street
Regina, Saskatchewan
S4P 1Y7

Volunteer Information Training Centre
No. 216
1933-8th Avenue
Regina, Saskatchewan
S4R 1E9

MANITOBA

CANADIAN ASSOCIATION FOR COMMUNITY LIVING

Association for Community Living
(Manitoba)
#1-90 Market Avenue
Winnipeg, Manitoba
R3B 0P3
947-1118

CANADIAN MENTAL HEALTH ASSOCIATION

Ms. Debbie Duprez
Branch Staff Contact
CMHA—Interlake Branch
c/o P.O. Box 11
Argyle, Manitoba
R0C 0B0

Mrs. Sally Cunningham
Branch Staff Contact
Canadian Mental Health Association
Westman Branch
935-26th Street
Brandon, Manitoba
R7B 2B7

Ms. Shirley Degryse
Community Coordinator
CMHA—Portage Branch
310 Princess Street
Portage La Prairie, Manitoba
R1N 0J9

Ms. Hazel Kent
Staff Contact
CMHA—Brokenhead Branch
Brokenhead Band Council
Scanterburry, Manitoba
R0E 1W0

Mr. Gordon Klassen
Staff Contact
CMHA—Steinbach Branch
P.O. Box 3699
Steinbach, Manitoba
R0A 2A0

Merle Dvorak
Branch Staff Contact
CMHA—Swan Valley Branch
Box 1755
Swan River, Manitoba
R0L 1Z0

Ms. Bev Gutray
Executive Director
CMHA—Winnipeg Branch
1-836 Ellice Avenue
Winnipeg, Manitoba
R3G 0C2

COMMUNITY SERVICES

Age and Opportunity
304-323 Portage Avenue
Winnipeg, Manitoba
R3B 2C1
947-1276

Bleak House Centre
1637 Main Street
Winnipeg, Manitoba
338-4723

Brandon Civic Senior Citizens Inc.
241-8th Street
Brandon, Manitoba
727-6641

Central
105-2nd Street
Morden, Manitoba
R0G 1J0
822-5425

Centre on Aging
338 Isbister Building
University of Manitoba
Winnipeg, Manitoba
R3T 2N2
474-8754

Eastman Region
20 1st Street
Beausejour, Manitoba
R0E 0C0
268-1411

Ellice Place
555 Ellice Avenue
Winnipeg, Manitoba
774-1110

Elmwood/East Kildonan Senior Centre
(sponsored by the City of Winnipeg)
180 Poplar at Brazier
Winnipeg, Manitoba
669-0750

Golden Age Club
1721 Main Street
Winnipeg, Manitoba
334-7362

Golden Rule Senior Centre
Fort Rouge Leisure Centre
625 Osborne Street
Winnipeg, Manitoba
452-5838

Gordon Howard Senior Centre
328 Vaughan Street
Selkirk, Manitoba
785-2092

Herman Prior Senior Centre
P.O. Box 1478
Portage la Prairie, Manitoba
857-6951

Immigrant Access Service
294 William Avenue
Winnipeg, Manitoba
R3B 0R1
945-6300

Interlake
202-446 Main Street
Selkirk, Manitoba
R1A 1V7
482-4511

Lions Place,
610 Portage Avenue
Winnipeg, Manitoba
775-8415

Main Street Senior Centre
817 Main Street
Winnipeg, Manitoba
942-5261

Meals on Wheels of Winnipeg Inc.
210-170 Marion Street
Winnipeg, Manitoba
R2H 0T4
233-8603

Norman Region
Box 2550
3rd Street
The Pas, Manitoba
R9A 1M4
623-6411

Program Directorate
Services to Seniors
4th Floor
831 Portage Avenue
Winnipeg, Manitoba
R3G 0N6

River Heights Senior Centre
1735 Corydon Avenue
Winnipeg, Manitoba
489-8040

Selkirk Avenue Senior Centre
460 Selkirk Avenue
Winnipeg, Manitoba
582-2329

Smith Street Senior Centre
2nd Floor
185 Smith Street
Winnipeg, Manitoba
942-6301

St. Boniface Senior Centre
817 Cathedral Avenue
Winnipeg, Manitoba
233-7973

St. Vital Senior Centre
613 St. Mary's Road
Winnipeg, Manitoba
253-1842

Stay Young Centre
Y.M.H.A. Jewish Community Centre
of Winnipeg
370 Hargrave Street
Winnipeg, Manitoba
947-0601

Stradbrook Senior Centre
400 Stradbrook Avenue
Winnipeg, Manitoba
475-9150

Support Services to Seniors
Coordinator
Manitoba Health
7th Floor
175 Hargrave Street
Winnipeg, Manitoba
R3C 3R8
945-8731

The Club
Lions Manor,
320 Sherbrook Street
Winnipeg, Manitoba
772-8887

West End Senior Centre
644 Brunell Street
Winnipeg, Manitoba
772-9581

Westman
340-9th Street
Brandon, Manitoba
R7A 2C6
726-6465

Winkler and District Senior Centre
Box 653
Winkler, Manitoba
R0G 2X0
325-8964

Winnipeg West
1981 Portage Avenue
Winnipeg, Manitoba
R3J 0J9
945-5850

Elsewhere in Manitoba for referral call:
Citizens' Inquiry Service:
1-800-282-8060

FAMILY SERVICE CANADA

Family Services of Winnipeg Inc.
400-287 Broadway
Winnipeg, Manitoba
R3C 0R9
204-947-1401

HEALTH, COMMUNITY SERVICES

Canadian Cancer Society
42 McTavish Avenue
Brandon, Manitoba
R7A 2B2
727-7577

Canadian Cancer Society
Box 873
Dauphin, Manitoba
R7N 3J5
638-8041

Canadian Cancer Society
Box 2128
Swan River, Manitoba
734-9260

Canadian Cancer Society
City Centre Mall
300 Mystery Lake Road
Thompson, Manitoba
R8N 0M2
677-5927

Canadian Cancer Society
193 Sherbrook
Winnipeg, Manitoba
R3C 2B7
744-7483

CNIB
356-10th Street
Brandon, Manitoba
R7A 4G1
727-0631

CNIB
1080 Portage Avenue
Winnipeg, Manitoba
R3G 3M3
774-5421

Canadian Paraplegic Association
825 Sherbrook Street
Winnipeg, Manitoba
R3A 1M5
786-4753

Central Region
25 Tupper Street N.
Portage la Prairie, Manitoba
R1N 3K1
857-9711

Community Therapy Services of
Manitoba
825 Sherbrook Street
Winnipeg, Manitoba
R3A 1M5
775-8657

Daily Hello
Winnipeg North 945-8333
Winnipeg South 945-8933
Winnipeg West 945-8911
Winnipeg Central 945-6333
or call
Citizen's Inquiry Service
945-3744
Toll free: 1-800-282-8060

Directory of Senior Citizen Residences
in Winnipeg
Age and Opportunity
304-323 Portage Avenue
Winnipeg, Manitoba
R3B 2C1
947-1276

Eastman Region
20 1st Street
Beausejour, Manitoba
R0E 0C0
268-1411

Health Action Centre
425 Elgin Avenue
Winnipeg, Manitoba
R3A 1P2
947-1626

Health Promotion Services
Nutrition: 945-8971
Services to Seniors: 945-6740
Fitness: 945-4404
or write to:
Manitoba Health
831 Portage Avenue
Winnipeg, Manitoba
R3G 0N6

The Independent Living
Resources Centre
207-294 Portage Avenue
Winnipeg, Manitoba
R3C 0B9

Interlake Region
202-446 Main Street
Selkirk, Manitoba
R1A 1V7
482-4511

Manitoba Federation of the
Visually Handicapped
200-294 Portage Avenue
Winnipeg, Manitoba
R3C 0B9
942-5895

Manitoba Heart Foundation
Box 33
203-42 McTavish Avenue E.
Brandon, Manitoba
R7A 5Y6
727-6971

Manitoba Heart Foundation
Box 873
Dauphin, Manitoba
R7N 3J5
638-8041

Manitoba Heart Foundation
Box 2128
Swan River, Manitoba
734-9260

Manitoba Heart Foundation
Canadian Cancer Society
City Centre Mall
300 Mystery Lake Road
Thompson, Manitoba
R8N 0M2
677-5927

Manitoba Heart Foundation
301-352 Donald Street
Winnipeg, Manitoba
R3B 2H8
942-0195

Manitoba Housing
287 Broadway Avenue
Winnipeg, Manitoba
R3C 0R9
945-4747

Manitoba League of the Physically
Handicapped, Inc.
200-294 Portage Avenue
Winnipeg, Manitoba
R3C 0B9
943-6099

Manitoba Telephone System
941-5735

Nor'West Co-op Health and Social
Services Centre Inc.
103-61 Tyndal Avenue
Winnipeg, Manitoba
R2X 2T4
633-5955

Norman Region
3rd and Ross Avenue
Box 2550
The Pas, Manitoba
R9A 1M4
623-6411

Office of the Ombudsman
Province of Manitoba
750-500 Portage Avenue
Winnipeg, Manitoba
R3C 3X1
786-6483

Parklands Region
15 1st Avenue S.W.
Dauphin, Manitoba
R7N 1R9
638-7024

Rupert's Land Respite Care
168 Wilton Street
Winnipeg, Manitoba
R3M 3C3
475-4031

Seniors Transport Service Inc.
1910 Pembina Highway
Winnipeg, Manitoba
R3T 4S5
269-2170
269-4080

Society for Manitobans with
Disabilities Inc.
825 Sherbrook Street
Winnipeg, Manitoba
(clients only)

Thompson Region
871 Thompson Drive
Thompson, Manitoba
R8N 0C8
778-7371

Victorian Order of Nurses
311-167 Lombard Avenue
Winnipeg, Manitoba
R3B 0T6
957-0650

The Volunteer Centre of Winnipeg
3rd Floor-5 Donald Street
Winnipeg, Manitoba
R3L 2T4
477-5180

Westman Region
340 9th Street
Brandon, Manitoba
R7A 6C2
726-6291

Winnipeg North
1021 Court Avenue
Winnipeg, Manitoba
R2P 1V7
945-8333

Winnipeg Public Library
Extension Library
1910 Portage Avenue
Winnipeg, Manitoba
R3J 0J2
832-0203

Winnipeg South
233 Provencher Blvd.
Winnipeg, Manitoba
R2H 0G4
945-8966

Winnipeg West and Central
189 Evanson Street
Winnipeg, Manitoba
R3G 0N9
945-6333

HOME SERVICES

Community Home Services, a project funded by the City of Winnipeg, provides a number of free services for low income senior citizens and disabled people throughout the city. They assist with house-cleaning, yard maintenance, snow shovelling, odd jobs of a non-technical nature, and one-way transportation to medical appointments.
Call 452-6735 or 475-6543
(Monday–Friday)

MEALS ON WHEELS

If your city is listed here, there is a Meals on Wheels program there. If there's no phone number listed, just look in your local telephone directory or ask any health professional in your area.

Altona, Manitoba
Arborg, Manitoba
Ashern, Manitoba
Baldur, Manitoba
Beausejour, Manitoba
Benito, Manitoba
Birtle, Manitoba
Boissevain, Manitoba
Brandon, Manitoba
Carberry, Manitoba
Carman, Manitoba
Cartwright, Manitoba
Cypress River, Manitoba
Dauphin, Manitoba
Deloraine, Manitoba
Dominion City, Manitoba
Elkhorn, Manitoba
Emerson, Manitoba
Ethelbert, Manitoba
Flin Flon, Manitoba
Foxwarren, Manitoba
Gilbert Plains, Manitoba
Glenboro, Manitoba
Grandview, Manitoba
Hamiota, Manitoba
Hartney, Manitoba

Holland, Manitoba
Ireherne, Manitoba
Kenton, Manitoba
Killarney, Manitoba
Lundar, Manitoba
MacGregor, Manitoba
Manitou, Manitoba
McAuley, Manitoba
McCreary, Manitoba
Melita, Manitoba
Minitonas, Manitoba
Minnedosa, Manitoba
Morden, Manitoba
Morris, Manitoba
Neepawa, Manitoba
Notre Dame de Loudres, Manitoba
Pine Falls, Manitoba
Portage la Prairie, Manitoba
Rathwell, Manitoba
Roblin, Manitoba
Rossburn, Manitoba
San Clara, Manitoba
Selkirk, Manitoba
Souris, Manitoba
St. Claude, Manitoba
Ste. Rose du Lac, Manitoba
Stonewall, Manitoba
Swan Lake, Manitoba
Swan River, Manitoba
Teulon, Manitoba
The Pas, Manitoba
Virden, Manitoba
Winkler, Manitoba
Winnipegosis, Manitoba

OCCUPATIONAL THERAPISTS

Association of Occupational Therapists of Manitoba (AOTM)
320 Sherbrook Street at Portage
Winnipeg, Manitoba
R3B 2W6
784-1272

Manitoba Society of Occupational
Therapists (MSOT)
884 William Avenue
Winnipeg, Manitoba
R3E 0Z6
774-4099

THE PARKINSON FOUNDATION
OF CANADA

Winnipeg, Manitoba
669-2130
476-7405

RED CROSS

Canadian Red Cross Society
Manitoba
226 Osborne Street North
Winnipeg, Manitoba
R3C 1V4
772-2551

SELF-HELP CLEARING HOUSES

Winnipeg Self Help Resource
Clearing House
NorWest Coop and Health Centre
103-61 Tyndall Avenue
Winnipeg, Manitoba
R2X 2T4
589-5500

SELF-HELP GROUPS

Age and Opportunity Centre
304-294 Portage Avenue
Winnipeg, Manitoba
R3C 0B9

Alzheimer Society of Manitoba Inc.
205 Edmonton Street
Winnipeg, Manitoba
R3C 1R4
943-6622

American Association of Marriage &
Family Therapists
c/o Interfaith Pastoral Institute
515 Portage Avenue
Winnipeg, Manitoba
R3B 2E9
269-8070 (home)/786-9160 (work)

The Arthritis Society
825 Sherbrook Street
Winnipeg, Manitoba
R3A 1M5
786-3486

Continuing Care—Home Care
Manitoba Health/Family Services
Eastman Region
20-1st Street
Box 50
Beausejour, Manitoba
R0E 0C0

Continuing Care—Home Care
Manitoba Health/Family Services
Westman Region
340-9th Street
Brandon, Manitoba

Continuing Care—Home Care
Manitoba Health/Family Services
Parklands Region
707-3rd Street, S.W.
Dauphin, Manitoba
R7N 1R8

Continuing Care—Home Care
Manitoba Health/Family Services
Central Region
25 Tupper Street North
Portage la Prairie, Manitoba
R1N 1W9

Continuing Care—Home Care
Manitoba Health/Family Services
Interlake Region
202-446 Main Street
Selkirk, Manitoba
R1A 1V7

Continuing Care—Home Care
Manitoba Health/Family Services
Norman Region
3rd and Ross Avenue
Box 2550
The Pas, Manitoba
R9A 1M4

Continuing Care—Home Care
Manitoba Health/Family Services
Thompson Region
871 Thompson Drive
Thompson, Manitoba
R8N 0C8

Continuing Care—Home Care
Manitoba Health/Family Services
1021 Court Avenue
Winnipeg, Manitoba
R2P 1V7

Continuing Care—Home Care
Manitoba Health/Family Services
233 Provencher Boulevard
Winnipeg, Manitoba
R2H 0G4

Continuing Care—Home Care
Manitoba Health/Family Services
Winnipeg West Central
189 Evanson Street
Winnipeg, Manitoba
R3G 0N9

Creative Retirement Manitoba
Brandon, Manitoba
726-4404

Creative Retirement Manitoba
Winnipeg, Manitoba
949-2565

Emergency Home Repair Program
(EHRP)
Winnipeg, Manitoba
945-2300/Toll Free 1-800-282-8069

Eye Glasses Program
Manitoba Health Services Commission
786-7101/Toll Free 1-800-392-1207

Family Services of Winnipeg Inc.
4th Floor
287 Broadway Avenue
Winnipeg, Manitoba
R3C 0R9
947-1401

Heart and Stroke Foundation of
Manitoba
301-352 Donald Street
Winnipeg, Manitoba
R3B 2H8
942-0195

Legal Aid Manitoba
Winnipeg, Manitoba
947-6501

Legal Aid Manitoba
Rural Manitoba
Citizen's Inquiry Service
Toll Free 1-800-282-8060

Legal Assistance
The Ombudsman
Winnipeg, Manitoba
795-6483/Toll Free 1-800-782-0394

Legal Services Information and Lawyer
Referral Program
Winnipeg, Manitoba
943-2305/Toll Free 1-800-262-8800

The Manitoba Chronic Pain
Association
P.O. Box 384
929 Corydon Avenue
Winnipeg, Manitoba
R3M 3V3
284-5909

Manitoba Council on Aging
(Handbook for Seniors)
Winnipeg, Manitoba
945-1997/Toll Free 1-800-665-6565

Manitoba Council on Aging
7th Floor
175 Hargrave Street
Winnipeg, Manitoba
R3C 3R8

Manitoba Society of Seniors
803 Somerset Place
294 Portage Avenue
Winnipeg, Manitoba
R3B 0B9
942-3147

Medication Information Line
for the Elderly
Faculty of Pharmacy
University of Manitoba
Winnipeg, Manitoba
261-3111/Rural Manitoba
Toll Free 1-800-432-1960, ext. 6493

Media
MSOS Journal
942-3147

MTS Special Needs Centre
904-294 Portage Avenue
Somerset Building
Winnipeg, Manitoba
941-8557

The Multiple Sclerosis Society
of Canada
Manitoba Division
825 Sherbrook Street
Winnipeg, Manitoba
R3A 1M5
783-8585

Personal Emergency Response
Seniors Directorate
Winnipeg, Manitoba
945-6565/Toll Free 1-800-665-6565

Pharmacare
at all drug stores
786-7141/Toll Free 1-800-392-1207

Program Directorate
Services to Seniors
302-333 Broadway Avenue
Winnipeg, Manitoba
R3C 0S9
945-6740

Provincial Gerontologist
Manitoba Health
7th Floor
175 Hargrave Street
Winnipeg, Manitoba
R3C 3R8

Regional Program Specialists
Eastman
20-1st Street
Beausejour, Manitoba
R0E 0C0
268-1411

Regional Program Specialists
Westman
340-9th Street
Brandon, Manitoba
R7A 2C6
726-6465

Regional Program Specialists
Parkland
707-3rd Street S.W.
Dauphin, Manitoba
R7N 1R8
638-7024

Regional Program Specialists
Central
105-2nd Street
Morden, Manitoba
R0G 1J0
822-5425

Regional Program Specialists
Interlake
202-446 Main Street
Selkirk, Manitoba
R1A 1V7

Regional Program Specialists
Norman
Box 2550
3rd Street
The Pas, Manitoba
R9A 1M4
623-6411

Regional Program Specialists
Winnipeg West
1981 Portage Avenue
Winnipeg, Manitoba
R3J 0J9
945-5850

Residential Rehabilitation Assistance
Program (RRAP)
Winnipeg, Manitoba
775-9561/Outside Winnipeg
1-800-542-3401/Rural 1-800-282-8069

Rural Handivan Program
Department of Highways and
Transportation
Winnipeg, Manitoba
945-2009/Toll Free 1-800-282-8069

Seniors Information Line
Toll Free: 1-800-665-6565

Seniors Outreach Office
Portage la Prairie, Manitoba
857-9711/Toll Free 1-800-665-0657

Seniors Outreach Office
The Pas, Manitoba
623-3085/Toll Free 1-800-665-0658

Media
Seniors Today
885-9700

Shelter Allowances for Elderly
Renters (SAFER)
Winnipeg, Manitoba
945-2611/Toll Free 1-800-282-8069

Societe Alzheimer Society
Suite B
170 Hargrave Street
Winnipeg, Manitoba
R3C 3H4
943-6622

The Stroke Assoc. of Manitoba Inc.
213-93 Lombard Avenue
Winnipeg, Manitoba
R3B 3B1
942-2880

Support Services to Seniors
Manitoba Health
302-333 Broadway Avenue
Winnipeg, Manitoba
R3C 0S9
945-8731

The Volunteer Centre Winnipeg
3rd floor
5 Donald
Winnipeg, Manitoba
R3L 2T4
477-5180

ONTARIO

CANADIAN ASSOCIATION FOR COMMUNITY LIVING

Ontario Association for
Community Living
1376 Bayview Avenue
Toronto, Ontario
M4G 3A3
(416) 483-4348

CANADIAN CANCER SOCIETY OFFICES

Metropolitan Toronto District Office
2 Carlton Street
Suite 710
Toronto, Ontario
M5B 2J2
(416) 593-1513

National Office
77 Bloor Street
Suite 1702
Toronto, Ontario
M5S 3A1

Ontario Division Office
1639 Yonge Street
Toronto, Ontario
M4T 2W6
(416) 488-5400

CANADIAN MENTAL HEALTH ASSOCIATION

Ms. Glenna Henderson
Executive Director
CMHA—Barrie Branch
17 Owen Street
3rd Floor
Barrie, Ontario
L4M 3G8

Mr. Roque Sager
Branch Staff Contact
CMHA—Hastings &
Prince Edward Counties
Box 1142
Belleville, Ontario
K8N 5B6

Mr. Ted van Overdijk
Executive Director
CMHA—Peel Region
34 Queen Street West
Brampton, Ontario
L6X 1A1

Ms. Peg Purvis
Executive Director
CMHA—Brant County Branch
21 Charlotte Street
Brantford, Ontario
N3T 2W3

Ms. Lynn Benoit
Executive Director
CMHA—Leeds/Grenville
58 King Street East
Brockville, Ontario
K6V 1B1

Mr. Derek Bishop
Chairperson
East Haldimand–Norfolk Steering
Committee
P.O. Box 749
Caledonia, Ontario
N0A 1A0

Ms. Barbara Garvin
Executive Director
CMHA—Kent County
93 William Street North
Chatham, Ontario
N7M 4L4

Ms. Carole Payer
Executive Director
CMHA—Cornwall, Stormont,
Dundas & Glengarry
29 Second Street East
Suite 5
Cornwall, Ontario
K6H 1Y2

Ms. Sheila Shaw
Executive Director
CMHA—Fort Frances
Box 446
Fort Frances, Ontario
P9A 3M8

Ms. Barbara Ancio
Chairperson
Huron County Steering Committee
P.O. Box 235
Goderich, Ontario
N7A 3Z2

Ms. Anne Vaughan
Executive Director
CMHA—Guelph/Wellington
421 Woolwich Street
Guelph, Ontario
N1H 3H2

Ms. Phyllis Turner
Executive Director
CMHA—Hamilton/Wentworth
1 Hunter Street East
Hamilton, Ontario
L8N 3W1

Mr. Larry Leafloor
Executive Director
CMHA—Kingston
388 King Street East
Kingston, Ontario
K7K 2Y2

Ms. Linda Ball
Director of Programming & Planning
P.O. Box 411
Kirkland Lake, Ontario
P2N 3J1

Ms. Marjorie Mank
Executive Director
CMHA—Waterloo Region
607 King Street West
Suite 202
Kitchener, Ontario
N2G 1C7

Ms. Donna Quance
Housing Coordinator
P.O. Box 1035
Lindsay, Ontario
K9V 5N4

Mike Petrenko
Executive Director
CMHA—London/Middlesex
355 Princess Avenue
London, Ontario
N6B 2A7

Ms. Carol J. West
Executive Director
CMHA—York Region
1111 Stellar Drive
Unit 4B
Newmarket, Ontario
L3Y 7B8

Mr. Richard Christie
Executive Director
CMHA—North Bay
240 Algonquin Avenue
Suite 304
North Bay, Ontario
P1B 4V9

Ms. Pearl Wolfe
Executive Director
CMHA—Oakville
341 Kerr Street
Oakville, Ontario
L6H 3B7

Ms. Linda Kydd
Executive Director
CMHA—Durham Region
111 Simcoe Street N.
Oshawa, Ontario
L1G 4S4

Ms. Barbara MacKinnon
Executive Director
CMHA—Ottawa/Carleton
44 Eccles Street
Ottawa, Ontario
K1R 6S4

Mr. Tom Jenks
Executive Director
CMHA—Grey Bruce County
1079 2nd Avenue East
Owen Sound, Ontario
N4K 2H8

Ms. Barbara Moffat
Executive Director
CMHA—Peterborough
P.O. Box 22
Peterborough, Ontario
K9J 9Y5

Ms. Kathy Janzen
Chairperson
West Haldimand–Norfolk
Steering Committee
P.O. Box 85
Port Dover, Ontario
N0A 1N0

Ms. Marilynne Ryan
Executive Director
Lochiel Kiwanis Centre
180 College Avenue North
3rd Floor
Sarnia, Ontario
N7T 7X7

Sister Leila Greco
Executive Director
CMHA—Sault Ste. Marie
120 Brock Street
Sault Ste. Marie, Ontario
P6A 3B5

Ms. Sheila Bristo
Executive Director
CMHA—St. Catharines & District
Branch
15 Wellington Street
St. Catharines, Ontario
L2R 5P7

Ms. Betty Couture
Executive Director
CMHA—Elgin County
P.O. Box 489
St. Thomas, Ontario
N5P 3V2

Ms. Marsha Stephen
Executive Director
CMHA—Perth County
380 Hibernia Street
Stratford, Ontario
N5A 5W3

Ms. Mary Ann Quinlan
Executive Director
CMHA—Sudbury Branch
111 Elm Street West
Sudbury, Ontario
P3C 1T3

Mr. Maurice Fortin
Executive Director
CMHA—Thunder Bay Branch
212 Camelot Street
Main Floor
Thunder Bay, Ontario
P7A 4B1

Ms. Judy Shanks
Executive Director
CMHA—Timmins Branch
239 Wilson Avenue
Timmins, Ontario
P4N 2T3

Mr. Steve Lurie
Executive Director
CMHA—Metro Toronto Branch
3101 Bathurst Street
5th Floor
Toronto, Ontario
M6A 2A6

Ms. Linda Hambling
Executive Director
CMHA—Welland
115 MacLean Place
Welland, Ontario
L3B 5X9

Ms. Pamela Hines
Executive Director
CMHA—Windsor/Essex
880 Ouellette Avenue
#901
Windsor, Ontario
N9A 1C7

Ms. Carole Nudds
Executive Director
CMHA—Oxford County
806 Dundas Street
Woodstock, Ontario
N4S 1G2

FAMILY SERVICE CANADA

Catholic Family Counselling Centre
74 Weber Street West
Kitchener, Ontario
N2H 3Z3
(519) 743-6333

Catholic Family Service Bureau
677 Victoria
Windsor, Ontario
N9A 4N3
(519) 254-5164

Catholic Family Service of Ottawa
200 Isabella Street
Ottawa, Ontario
K1S 1V7
(613) 233-8478

Catholic Family Services of
Hamilton–Wentworth
82 Stinson Street
Hamilton, Ontario
L8N 1S2
(416) 527-3823

Catholic Family Services of Toronto
67 Bond Street
Toronto, Ontario
M5B 1X5
(416) 362-2481

Catholic Social Services
562 Wellington Street
London, Ontario
N6A 3R5
(519) 432-4107

Family Counselling Centre
681 Oxford Street
Sarnia, Ontario
N7T 6Z7
(519) 336-0120

Family Counselling Service of Kingston
388 King Street East
Kingston, Ontario
K7K 2Y2
(613) 549-7850

Family Day Care Services
380 Sherbourne Street
Toronto, Ontario
M4X 1K2
(416) 922-9556

The Family Service Bureau of Windsor
and Essex County
450 Victoria Avenue
Windsor, Ontario
N9A 6T7
(519) 256-1831

The Family Service Centre of
Ottawa–Carleton
119 Ross Avenue
Ottawa, Ontario
K1Y 0N6
(613) 725-3601

Family Service London
90 Albert Street
London, Ontario
N6A 1L8
(519) 433-0183

Family Services Centre of
Sault Ste. Marie and District
421 Bay Street
Suite 603
Sault Ste. Marie, Ontario
P6A 1X3
(705) 759-2756

Family Services for
Southwest York Region
10225A Yonge Street
P.O. Box 244
Richmond Hill, Ontario
L4C 4Y2
(416) 884-9148

Family Services of
Hamilton–Wentworth Inc.
350 King Street East
Suite 201
Hamilton, Ontario
L8N 3Y3
(416) 523-5640

Family Services of
Metropolitan Toronto
22 Wellesley Street East
Toronto, Ontario
M4Y 1G3
(416) 922-3126

Family Services of Peel
P.O. Box 310
Postal Station A
151 City Centre Drive
Mississauga, Ontario
L5A 3A1
(416) 270-2250

Family Services Thunder Bay
411 Donald Street East
Thunder Bay, Ontario
P7E 5V1
(807) 623-9596

Halton Family Services
235 Lakeshore Road East
P.O. Box 671
Oakville, Ontario
L6J 5C1
(416) 845-3811

The Regional Municipality of Durham
Social Services Department
50 McMillan Drive
Oshawa, Ontario
L1G 3Z6
(416) 579-0622

Service Familial de Sudbury/
Sudbury Family Service
45 rue Elm Street East
Sudbury, Ontario
P3C 1S2
(705) 674-5456

Social Planning and Research Council
of Hamilton and District
155 James Street S.
Suite 602
Hamilton, Ontario
L8P 3A4
(416) 522-1148

Social Planning Council of
Ajax–Pickering
132A Commercial Avenue
Ajax, Ontario
L1S 2H5
(416) 686-2661

MEALS ON WHEELS

*If your city is listed here, there is a
Meals on Wheels program there. If
there's no phone number listed, just
look in your local telephone directory
or ask any health professional in your
area.*

Acton, (519) 853-3310

Alliston, (705) 424-1509

Angus, (705) 424-1509

Atikokan, (807) 597-6295

Aurora

Aylmer West

Bala, (705) 762-3740

Bancroft, (613) 332-4700

Barrie, (705) 728-7220

Beamsville, (416) 563-7449

Beeton, (705) 729-2267

Belleville, (613) 969-0130

Blind River, (705) 356-9860

Bobcaygeon

Bolton, (416) 857-3806

Bradford, (416) 750-3517

Brampton, (416) 459-3333
(416) 453-4140

Brantford, (519) 753-4188

Brockville, (613) 342-2251

Burford, (519) 449-5106

Burks Falls, (705) 382-2905

Burlington, (416) 637-5664

Caledonia, (416) 765-6892

Cambridge, (519) 653-5427
(519) 521-8120
(519) 740-3235

Campbellford, (705) 653-1140

Chatham

Chesley

Chesterville, (613) 448-2674

Cobourg, (416) 372-7356

Cochenour, (807) 662-8131

Colborne, (416) 324-7323

Collingwood, (705) 445-5577

Cornwall, (613) 933-4320

Deep River, (613) 584-4316

Delhi, (519) 582 0290
(519) 582 1370

Don Mills, (416) 447-7244

Dorchester, (519) 451-8523

Dryden

Dundalk

Dunnville, (416) 774-3547

Durham

Elliot Lake, (705) 848-2285

Elmira

Elmvale

Elora

Emo, (807) 482-2207

Erin, (519) 833-2312

Espanola, (705) 869-1420

Essex, (519) 776-6689

Fenelon Falls

Fergus

Fort Francis, (807) 274-3379

Georgetown

Grand Valley

Gravenhurst, (705) 687-6988

Grimsby, (416) 945-5135

Guelph, (519) 822-8441

Hagersville, (519) 768-5588

Haliburton, (705) 457-2942/2171

Hamilton, (416) 522-1022
(416) 575-1500

Hanover, (519) 364-2340

Harriston, (519) 338-2190

Hawkesbury, (613) 632-2095

Hornepayne, (807)868-2442

Huntsville

Iroquois Falls, (705) 258-3836

Kenora, (807)468-3156

Kincardine, (519) 396-3138

King City

Kingston, (613) 354-3301

Kirkland Lake, (705) 567-7383

Kitchener, (519) 743-8671

Lakefield

Lindsay, (705) 324-8323

Lion's Head, (519) 534-2893

Listowel, (519) 291-2053

Little Britain

London, (519) 439-0607

Lucknow

Markdale

Midland, (705) 526-9333

Millbrook

Milton, (416) 878-6639

Mississauga, (416) 823-1460
(416) 275-2860

Mitchell, (519) 348-9535

Morpeth

Morrisburg, (613) 543-3422

Mount Albert

Mount Forest, (519) 323-2210

Napanee, (613) 354-3301

Nepean, (613) 828-3362

New Hamburg

River Drive Park
Meals On Wheels
Newmarket

Newmarket, (416) 764-5946

Niagara Falls, (416) 468-3676

Niagara-on-the-Lake, (416) 468-3676

Nobleton

Noelville, (705) 898-2174

North Bay, (705) 472-2855

North York, (416) 635-2860
(416) 633-9519

Oakville, (416) 842-1411

Orangeville

Orillia, (705) 325-9845

Orono

Oshawa, (416) 723-2933

Ottawa, (613) 235-0000
(613) 233-2424

Owen Sound, (519) 376-1707

Paris, (519) 442-3242

Parry Sound

Penetanguishene, (705) 549-7431

Peterborough, (705) 749-0200
(705) 745-5522

Petrolia, (519) 882-1068

Pickering, (416) 683-6141

Picton, (613) 476-7493

Port Colborne, (416) 835-5228

Port Dover, (519) 583-2335

Port Elgin

Port Hope, (416) 885-9710

Port Lambton

Rainy River, (807) 852-4450
(807) 852-3872

Red Rock, (807) 886-2895

Richmond Hill, (416) 883-1789

Ridgetown

Ridgeway, (416) 894-2015

Rockwood

Sarnia, (519) 337-2994

Sault Ste. Marie, (705) 942-2204

Scarborough, (416) 694-1138
(416) 439-5012

Schomberg, (416) 939-7128

Shelbourne, (519) 925-3794

Shelburne

Simcoe, (519) 426-0750 ext. 246

Sioux Lookout, (807) 737-3142
(807) 737-1723

Southampton

St. Catharines, (416) 641-2050

St. George, (519) 448-1120

St. Marys, (519) 284-3425

St. Thomas

St. Williams, (519) 586-3331

Stayner

Stratford, (519) 271-4692

Stroud, (705)436-5992

Sudbury, (705) 675-3338

Teeswater, (519) 392-6888

Terrace Bay, (807) 825-3273 ext. 192

Thornbury, (519) 599-3940

Thornhill, (416) 881-0917

Thorold, (416) 227-1360

Thunder Bay, (807) 622-6322

Tillsonburg, (519) 842-9517

Timmins, (705) 257-4900

Toronto, (416) 532-3657
(416) 366-3571
(416) 789-2113 ext.45
(416) 532-2202
(416) 424-3322
(416) 236-1056
(416) 466-0587
(416) 929-0811
(416) 481-6411
(416) 657-1204
(416) 962-9449

Trenton, (613) 392-5971

Tweed, (613) 478-5626

Vineland Stn., (416) 563-8252
(416) 562-4348

Walkerton

Wallaceburg, (519) 627-6208

Wardsville, (519) 693-4903

Waterdown

Waterford, (519) 443-7753

Wawa, (705) 856-2335

Welland, (416) 788-3181

Wellesley

West Hill, (416) 284-5931

Weston, (416) 249-7946

Whitby, (416) 668-6583

Wiarton

Willowdale, (416) 756-6042

Windsor, (519) 253-4211

Woodstock, (519) 539-1233

OCCUPATIONAL THERAPISTS

Ontario College of Occupational
Therapists (OCOT)
801 Eglinton Avenue West
Suite 200
Toronto, Ontario
M5N 1E3
781-7815

Ontario Society of Occupational
Therapists (OSOT)
781-8290

THE PARKINSON FOUNDATION OF CANADA

Ajax, (416) 683-0336

Amhurstville, (613) 389-1130

Belfountain, (519) 927-3204

Belleville, (613) 968-6467

Brechin, (705) 484-1318

Camlachie, (519) 869-4750

Chatham, (519) 354-2437
(519) 354-9951

Cornwall, 902-675-2416

Delhi, (519) 582-0585

Don Mills, (416) 441-1890

Guelph, (519) 824-1241

Hamilton, (416) 527-3655

Kingston, (613) 389-4820
(613) 546-2175

Kitchener, (519) 576-3320
(519) 579-1433

Lakefield, (705) 652-7401

London, (519) 672-6492
(519) 685-8500
(519) 439-9088
(519) 438-0086
(519) 471-3435

Mississauga, (416) 276-8346

Niagara Falls, (416) 354-9051

Oakville, (416) 842-2439
(416) 844-8992

Orillia, (705) 326-2832

Penticton, (604) 492-8505

Peterborough, (705) 742-0733

Sault Ste. Marie, (705) 254-7718
(705) 942-4989
(705) 253-4935

Shelburne, (519) 925-2375

Smiths Falls, (613) 283-6745
(613) 283-2504

St. Catharines, (416) 684-5320

Strathroy, (519) 586-4644

Whitby, (416) 666-8657

Willowdale, (416) 250-8141
(416) 483-7994

Woodstock, (519) 537-5956

RED CROSS

Canadian Red Cross Society
Ontario
5700 Cancross Court
Mississauga, Ontario
L5R 3E9

SELF-HELP CLEARING HOUSES

Canadian Council on Social
Development
P.O. Box 3505
Station C
Ottawa, Ontario
K1Y 4G1
(613) 728-1865

SELF-HELP GROUPS

Ajax, Pickering & Whitby Association
for Community Living
Pine Ridge Council
50 Commercial Street
#212
Ajax, Ontario
L1S 2H5
(416) 427-3300

Almaguin Highlands
Community Living
North Central Ontario Council
P.O. Box #370
Sundridge, Ontario
P0A 1Z0
(705) 384-5383

American Association of Marriage &
Family Therapists
Suite 15A
2 Orchard Heights Boulevard
Aurora, Ontario
L4G 3W3
(416) 841-3173 (home)
(416) 841-6565 (work)

Arnprior District Association for
Community Living
Champlain Council
P.O. Box #210
Braeside, Ontario
(613) 623-5830

Atikokan & District Association for the
Mentally Retarded
Northwestern Ontario Council
P.O. Box #2054
Atikokan, Ontario
P0T 1C0
(807) 597-2259

Barrie & District Association for
People with Special Needs
Simcoe County Regional Council
P.O. Box #1017
Barrie, Ontario
L4M 5E1
(705) 726-9082

Belleville & District Association for the
Mentally Retarded
Algoma Council
P.O. Box #70
Blind River, Ontario
P0R 1B0
(705) 356-7760

Brampton–Caledon Association for the
Mentally Retarded
Peel, Halton, Dufferin
Regional Council
220 Rutherford Road South
Brampton, Ontario
L6W 3J6
(416) 453-8833

Brantford and District Association for
Community Living
Hamilton–Lake Erie Council on
Mental Retardation
20 Bell Lane
R.R. #2
Brantford, Ontario
N3T 5L5
(519) 756-2662

Brockville & District Association for
Community Involvement
Thousand Island Council
P.O. Box #423
Brockville, Ontario
K6V 5V6
(613) 345-4092

Burlington Association for
Community Living
Peel, Halton, Dufferin Regional
Council
831 Legion Road
Burlington, Ontario
L77S 1T6
(416) 681-0393

Burlington Volunteer Centre
Suite 406B
760 Brant Street
Burlington, Ontario
L7R 4B7
(416) 639-4804

Cambridge & District Association for
the Mentally Handicapped
Wellington–Waterloo Council
60 Kerr Street
Cambridge, Ontario
N1R 4A3
(519) 623-7490

Cambridge Volunteer Bureau
2nd Floor
Dickson Centre
30 Parkhill Road West
Cambridge, Ontario
N1C 1C9
(519) 623-0423

Central Volunteer Bureau
Belleville Inc.
240 William Street
Belleville, Ontario
K8N 3K3
(613) 969-8862

Central Volunteer Bureau
2nd Floor
415 Dundas Street
London, Ontario
N6B 1V9
(519) 438-4155

Collingwood Community Living
Simcoe County Regional Council
3 Ronell Crescent
Collingwood, Ontario
L9Y 4J6
(705) 445-6351

Community Living Association for
South Simcoe
Simcoe County Regional Council
P.O. Box #100
Alliston, Ontario
L0M 1A0
(705) 435-4792

Community Living Association
(Lanark County)
Thousand Islands Council
178 Townline Road
Carleton Place, Ontario
K7C 2C2
(613) 257-8040

Community Living Central Huron
Midwestern Ontario Council
P.O. Box 527
Goderich, Ontario
N7A 4C7
(519) 524-7363

Community Living Fort Erie
Niagara Regional Council
P.O. Box #225
615 Industrial Avenue
Fort Erie, Ontario
L2A 5M9
(416) 871-6770

Community Living Huntsville
North Central Ontario Council
P.O. Box #2910
Huntsville, Ontario
P0A 1K0
(705) 789-4543

Community Living Huronia
Simcoe County Regional Council
P.O. Box #651
Midland, Ontario
L4R 4P4
(705) 526-4253

Community Living Kincardine
& District
Georgian Bay Council
P.O. Box #9000
Kincardine, Ontario
N2Z 2X8
(519) 396-9434

Community Living Mississauga
Peel, Halton, Dufferin Regional
Council
2444 Hurontario Street
3rd floor
Mississauga, Ontario
L5B 2V1
(416) 566-1365

Community Living Niagara Falls
Niagara Regional Council
4609 Crysler Avenue
Niagara Falls, Ontario
L2E 3V6
(416) 357-5605

Community Living Owen Sound
and District
Georgian Bay Council
259 8th Street East (upstairs)
Owen Sound, Ontario
N4K 1L2
(519) 371-9251

Community Living Renfrew & District
Champlain Council
P.O. Box #683
Renfrew, Ontario
K7V 4E7
(519) 371-9251

Community Living South Muskoka
North Central Ontario Council
P.O. Box #1271
Bracebridge, Ontario
P0B 1C0
(705) 645-5494

Community Living Stormont County
Eastern Ontario Council
812 Pitt Street North
Box 1B1
Cornwall, Ontario
K6J 5R4
(613) 938-1702

Community Living Timmins
Integration Communautaire
Northeastern Council
223 Third Avenue
Timmins, Ontario
P4N 1C9
(705) 268-8811

Community Living Wiarton & District
Georgian Bay Council
P.O. Box #95
Wiarton, Ontario
N0H 2T0
(519) 534-0918

Dryden Association for
Community Living
Northwestern Ontario Council
P.O. Box #329
Dryden, Ontario
P8N 2Z1
(807) 223-6160

Dryden Volunteer Bureau
4 Earl Avenue
Dryden, Ontario
P8N 1X3
(807) 233-5995

Dufferin Association for
Community Living
Peel, Halton, Dufferin Regional
Council
14 Stewart Court, #100
Orangeville, Ontario
L9W 3Z9
(519) 941-8971

Dundas County Association for the
Mentally Retarded
Eastern Ontario Council
P.O. Box 678
Morrisburg, Ontario
K0C 1X0
(613) 543-3737

Elliot Lake & District Association for
the Mentally Retarded
Algoma Council
P.O. Box #74
Elliot Lake, Ontario
P5A 2J6
(705) 848-2562

Elmira & District Association
for the Retarded
Wellington–Waterloo Council
158 Church Street West
Elmira, Ontario
N3B 1N3
(519) 669-1567

Espanola & District Association for
Community Living
Sudbury & Manitoulin Council
P.O. Box #1398
Espanola, Ontario
P0P 1C0

Essex County Association for
Community Living
Lake St. Clair Council
49 Talbot Street North
Essex, Ontario
N8M 1A3
(519) 776-6485

Fort Frances & District Association for
the Mentally Retarded
Northwestern Council
P.O. Box #147
Fort Frances, Ontario
P9A 3M5
(807) 274-5556

Fort Frances Volunteer Bureau
428 Victoria Avenue
Fort Frances, Ontario
P9A 2C3
(807) 274-9555

Gananoque & District Association for
the Mentally Retarded
Thousand Islands Council
The Barriefield
R.R. #2, Unit #407
Kingston, Ontario
K7L 5H7
(613) 549-2006

Georgina Association for
Community Living
York Council
P.O. Box #68
Sutton West, Ontario
L0E 1R0
(416) 722-8468/8947

Geraldton & District Association for
the Mentally Retarded
Lake Superior Council
P.O. Box #970
Geraldton, Ontario
P0T 1M0
(807) 854-0775

Glengarry Association for
Community Living
Eastern Council
P.O. Box #1659
Alexandria, Ontario
K0C 1A0
(613) 525-4357

Grimsby/Lincoln & District
Association for Community Living Inc.
Niagara Regional Council
P.O. Box #220
Beamsville, Ontario
L0R 1B0
(416) 563-4123/4115

Guelph Wellington Association for
Community Living
Wellington–Waterloo Council
319 Speedvale Avenue East
Guelph, Ontario
N1E 1N4
(519) 824-2480

Haldimand Association for the
Mentally Retarded
(Hamilton–Lake Erie Council)
P.O. Box #396
Cayuga, Ontario
N0A 1E0
(416) 772-3344

Haliburton & District Association for
the Mentally Retarded
Pine Ridge Council
P.O. Box #90
Haliburton, Ontario
K0M 1S0
(705) 457-2626

Halton Hills Volunteer Centre
Suite 10
164 Guelph Street
Georgetown, Ontario
L7G 4A6
(416) 877-3219

Hamilton & District Association for
the Mentally Retarded
Hamilton–Lake Erie Council
191 York Blvd.
Hamilton, Ontario
L8R 1Y6
(416) 528-0281

Hearst & District Association for the
Mentally Retarded
Northeastern Ontario Council
P.O. Box #7000
Hearst, Ontario
P0L 1N0
(705) 362-5758

Helpmate Volunteer Bureau
M. L. McConaghy Centre
Suite 309
10100 Yonge Street
Richmond Hill, Ontario
L4C 1T8
(416) 884-3839

Information Sudbury
Suite 208
109 Elm Street
Sudbury, Ontario
P3C 1T4
(705) 674-4636

Integration Communautaire Chapleau
Community Living
Sudbury & Manitoulin Council
P.O Box #1377
Chapleau, Ontario
P0M 1K0

Integration Communautaire Cochrane
Association for Community Living
Northeastern Ontario Council
P.O. Box #2330
Cochrane, Ontario
P0L 1C0
(705) 272-3853

Iroquois Falls Association for
Community Living
Northeastern Ontario Council
P.O. Box #1180
Iroquois Falls, Ontario
P0K 1G0
(705) 232-4490

K–W Association for Community
Living
Wellington–Waterloo Council
26 College Street
Kitchener, Ontario
N2H 4Z9
(519) 743-5783

Kapuskasing & District Association for
Community Living
Northeastern Ontario Council
12 Kimberley Drive
Kapuskasing, Ontario
P5N 1L5
(705) 337-1417

Kenora Association for
Community Living
Northwestern Ontario Council
501 8th Avenue South
Kenora, Ontario
P9N 3Z9
(807) 468-3161

Kingston & District Association for
Community Living
Thousand Islands Council
178 Sydenham Street
P.O. Box #1312
Kingston, Ontario
K7L 4Y8
(613) 546-6613

Kingston Community Volunteer Bureau
23 Carlisle Street
Kingston, Ontario
K7K 3X1
(613) 542-8512

Kirkland Lake & District Association
for the Mentally Retarded
Northeastern Ontario Council
23 Government Road West
Kirkland Lake, Ontario
P2N 3M7
(705) 567-6525

Lakehead Association for
Community Living
Lake Superior Council
521 Memorial Avenue
Thunder Bay, Ontario
P7B 3Y6
(807) 344-5761

Lambton County Association for the
Mentally Handicapped
Lake St. Clair Council
339 Centre Street, Box #569
Petrolia, Ontario
N0N 1R0
(519) 882-0933

Lennox & Addington Association for
the Mentally Retarded
Lake Ontario Council
P.O. Box #303
Napanee, Ontario
K7R 3M4
(613) 354-2184

Listowel & District Association for
Community Living
Midwestern Ontario Council
124 Davidson Avenue South
Listowel, Ontario
N4W 2J6
(519) 291-5581

London & District Association for the
Mentally Retarded
Midwestern Regional Council
190 Adelaide Street South
London, Ontario
N5Z 3L1
(519) 686-3000

Madawaska Valley Association for
Community Living
Champlain Council
P.O. Box #338
Barry's Bay, Ontario
K0J 1B0
(613) 756-3817

Manitoulin District Association for the
Mentally Retarded
Sudbury & Manitoulin Council
P.O. Box #152
Mindemoya, Ontario
(705) 377-6699

Marathon/Schreiber–Terrace Bay &
District Association for the
Mentally Retarded
Lake Superior Council
P.O. Box #550
P0T 2E0
(807) 229-2577

Markham Volunteer Bureau
5871 Highway #7
Markham, Ontario
L3P 1A3
(416) 471-1620

Meaford & District Association for the
Mentally Retarded
Georgian Bay Council
P.O. Box #44
Meaford, Ontario
N0H 1Y0

Milton Volunteer Centre
311 Commercial Street
Milton, Ontario
L9T 3Z9
(416) 876-4756

Moosonee–Moose Factory Association
for the Mentally Retarded
Northeastern Ontario Council
P.O. Box #460
Moosonee, Ontario
P0L 1Y0
(705) 336-2967

Newmarket & District Association for
Community Living
York Council
757 Bogart Avenue
Newmarket, Ontario
L3Y 2A7
(416) 898-3000
(416) 773-3613 (Toronto)

Niagara Falls Volunteer Bureau
5017 Victoria Avenue
Niagara Falls, Ontario
L2E 4C9
(416) 357-0300

Nipigon, Red Rock & District
Association for Community Living
Lake Superior Council
P.O. Box #918
Nipigon, Ontario
P0T 2J0
(807) 887-2835

Noelville & District Association
for the Handicapped &
Mentally Retarded
Sudbury & Manitoulin Council
R. R. #1
St. Charles, Ontario
P0M 2W0
(705) 867-2827

Norfolk Association for
Community Living
Hamilton–Lake Erie Council
139 Colborne Street South
Simcoe, Ontario
N3Y 4H4
(519) 426-5000

North Bay & District Association for
the Mentally Retarded
North Central Ontario Council
161 Main Street East
North Bay, Ontario
P1B 1A9
(705) 476-3288

North Frontenac, Ontario
Thousand Islands Council
P.O. Box #76
Sharbot Lake, Ontario
K0H 2P0
(613) 335-2120

North Grenville Association for
Community Living
Thousand Islands Council
P.O. Box #1430
Kemptville, Ontario
K0G 1J0
(613) 258-7177

North Halton Association for the
Developmentally Handicapped
Peel, Halton, Dufferin
Regional Council
62 Park Avenue
Georgetown, Ontario
L7G 4Z1
(416) 877-5557

North Hastings Community
Integration Association
Lake Ontario Council
P.O. Box #1508
Bancroft, Ontario
(613) 332-1310

North Wentworth Association for the
Mentally Retarded Inc.
Hamilton–Lake Erie Council
459 Ofield Road South
R.R. #2
Dundas, Ontario
L9H 5E2
(416) 628-6147

Northumberland Volunteer
Bureau/Centre
Post Office Box 7
R.R. #2
Roseneath, Ontario
K0K 2X0

Oakville Association for the
Mentally Retarded
Peel, Halton, Dufferin Regional
Council
1108 Speers Road
Oakville, Ontario
L6L 2Z4
(416) 844-0146

Oakville Volunteer Centre
2nd Floor
341 Kerr Street
Oakville, Ontario
L6K 3B7
(416) 849-8163

Ontario March of Dimes
Outreach Attendant Care
P.O. Box 1999
Brockville, Ontario
K6V 2G5
(613) 342-1935

Ontario March of Dimes
Outreach Attendant Care
Algo Centre
151 Ibtarui Avenue
Elliot Lake, Ontario
P6A 6L7
(705) 848-4840

Ontario March of Dimes
Outreach Attendant Care
20 Emerald Street North
Hamilton, Ontario
L8L 8A4
(416) 527-6653

Ontario March of Dimes
Outreach Attendant Care
311 Commercial Street
Milton, Ontario
L9T 3Z9
(416) 876-4466

Ontario March of Dimes
Outreach Attendant Care
202-3034 Palstan Road
Mississauga, Ontario
L4Y 2Z6
(416) 276-6252

Ontario March of Dimes
Outreach Attendant Care
Unit 2
165 Main Street South
Mount Forest, Ontario
N0G 2L0
(519) 323-1382

Ontario March of Dimes
Outreach Attendant Care
80 Colonnade Road
Nepean, Ontario
K2E 7L2
(613) 225-4765

Ontario March of Dimes
Outreach Attendant Care
180 Main Street South
Newmarket, Ontario
L3Y 3Z2
(416) 853-0383

Ontario March of Dimes
Outreach Attendant Care
3300 Merrittville Highway
P.O. Box 128
Thorold, Ontario
L2V 3Y7
(416) 687-8484

Ontario March of Dimes
Ridley Terrace
Apartment 101-103
448 Louth Street
St. Catharines, Ontario
L2S 3S9
(416) 641-4911

Ontario March of Dimes
SSLU and Outreach Attendant Care
Unit 104
15 Keil Drive North
Chatham, Ontario
N7L 1C5
(519) 351-8464

Ontario March of Dimes
SSLU and Outreach Attendant Care
507 Louisa Street
Point Edward, Ontario
N7V 3V8
(519) 332-4702

Ontario March of Dimes
Support Service Living Unit
309-20 Emerald Street North
Hamilton, Ontario
L8L 8A4
(416) 527-6653

Ontario March of Dimes
Support Service Living Unit
Apartment 102
Britannia Place
25 Glen Hawthorne Boulevard
Mississauga, Ontario
L5R 3E6
(416) 568-2410

Ontario March of Dimes
Support Service Living Unit
112-700 Bay Street
Sault Ste. Marie, Ontario
P6A 6L7
(705) 759-0328

Ontario March of Dimes
Villa Verdi
20 Jarvis Street
Hamilton, Ontario
L8R 1M2
(416) 528-4261

Orillia Association for the
Handicapped
Simcoe County Regional Council
6 Kitchener Street
Orillia, Ontario
L3V 6Z9
(705) 327-5391

Oshawa & District Association for
Community Living
Pine Ridge Council
39 Wellington Street East
Oshawa, Ontario
L1H 3Y1
(416) 576-3011

Pembroke & District Association for
Community Living
Champlain Council
P.O. Box #1030
Pembroke, Ontario
K8A 6Y6
(613) 735-0659

Peterborough & District Association
for Community Living
Pine Ridge Council
277 George Street North
P.O. Box #269
Peterborough, Ontario
K9J 6Y8
(705) 743-2411

Peterborough & District Information
Centre and Volunteer Bureau
229 King Street
Peterborough, Ontario
K9J 2R8
(705) 743-2523

Port Colborne District Association for
Community Living, Inc.
Niagara Regional Council
P.O. Box #579
Port Colborne, Ontario
L3K 5X8
(416) 835-8941

Port Hope–Cobourg & District
Association for Community Living
Pine Ridge Council
P.O. Box #835
Cobourg, Ontario
K9A 4S3
(416) 372-4455

Prescott & Russell Association for the
Mentally Retarded
Eastern Ontario Council
207 rue William Street, #5
Hawkesbury, Ontario
K6A 1X2
(613) 632-8536

Prince Edward Association for the
Mentally Retarded
Lake Ontario Council
P.O. Box #2409
Picton, Ontario
K0K 2T0
(613) 476-6038

Quad County Association for the
Mentally Retarded
Midwestern Ontario Council
P.O. Box #65
Wardsville, Ontario
N0L 2N0
(519) 693-4812

Red Lake & District Association for the
Mentally Retarded
Northwestern Ontario Council
P.O. Box #30
Red Lake, Ontario
P0V 2M0
(807) 749-2431

Ms. Denise Lauzon-Leblanc
Reseau Action Benevole
331 rue McGill
Hawkesbury, Ontario
K6A 1P9

Sarnia & District Association for
Community Living
Lake St. Clair Council
P.O. Box #610
551 Exmouth Street, #202
Sarnia, Ontario
N7T 7J4
(519) 332-0560

Saugeen Association for the
Mentally Retarded
Georgian Bay Council
P.O. Box #1810
Pt. Elgin, Ontario
N0H 2C0

Sault Ste. Marie Association for
Community Living
Algoma Council
96 White Oak Drive East
Sault Ste. Marie, Ontario
P6B 4J8
(705) 946-1234

Sioux Lookout-Hudson Association for
Community Living
Northwestern Ontario Council
P.O. Box #546
Sioux Lookout, Ontario
P0V 2T0

South Huron & District Association for
the Mentally Handicapped
Midwestern Ontario Council
P.O. Box #29
Dashwood, Ontario
N0M 1N0
(519) 237-3637

South West Grey Association for
Community Living
Georgian Bay Council
P.O. Box #645
Durham, Ontario
N0G 1R0
(519) 369-2181

South-East Grey Support Services
Georgian Bay Council
75 Main Street West
Markdale, Ontario
N0C 1H0
(519) 986-3220

St. Catharines Association for
Community Living
Niagara Regional Council
437 Welland Avenue
St. Catharines, Ontario
L2M 5Z6
(416) 688-5222

St. Marys Association for
Community Development
Midwestern Ontario Council
P.O. Box #1618
St. Marys, Ontario
N0M 2V0
(519) 284-1400

St. Thomas–Elgin Association for
Community Living
Midwestern Ontario Council
544 Talbot Street
St. Thomas, Ontario
N5P 1C4
(519) 631-9222

Stratford Area Association for
Community Living
Midwestern Ontario Council
379 Huron Street
Stratford, Ontario
N5A 5T6
(519) 273-1000

Strathroy and Area Association for
Community Living
Midwestern Ontario Council
71 Frank Street
P.O. Box #276
Strathroy, Ontario
N7G 3J2
(519) 245-5654

Sudbury & District Association for
Community Living
Sudbury & Manitoulin Council
P.O. Box #788
Station B
Sudbury, Ontario
P3E 4S1
(705) 674-1451

Tillsonburg & District Association for
Community Living
Midwestern Ontario Council
19 Queen Street
Tillsonburg, Ontario
N4G 3G5
(519) 842-6481

Timmins Volunteer Centre Inc.
Suite #1
251-3rd Avenue
Timmins, Ontario
P4N 1W2
(705) 264-9765

Trenton–Brighton & District
Association for the Mentally Retarded
Lake Ontario Council
11 Canal Street
Trenton, Ontario
K8V 4K3
(613) 394-2222

Tri-Municipal Volunteer Bureau
Corner 2nd Avenue and Fifth Street
P.O. Box 3011
Kenora, Ontario
P9N 3X4
(807) 468-5848

Tri-Town & District Association for
Community Living
Northeastern Ontario Council
P.O. Box #1149
Haileybury, Ontario
P0J 1K0
(705) 672-2000

Valley Association for Community
Living/Integration Communautaire
Sudbury & Manitoulin Council
P.O. Box #457
Val Caron, Ontario
P0M 3A0
(705) 897-6752

Victoria County Association for
Community Living
Pine Ridge Council
14 Lindsay Street North
P.O. Box 84
Lindsay, Ontario
K9V 4R8
(705) 328-0464

Voluntary Action Centre
of Hamilton & District
Suite 206
625 Main Street East
Hamilton, Ontario
L8M 1J5
(416) 529-4202

Voluntary Action Centre
of Thunder Bay
Suite 116
105 North May Street
Thunder Bay, Ontario
P7C 3N9
(705) 623-8272

Volunteer Brant
Suite 204
233 Colborne Street
P.O. 2108
Brantford, Ontario
N3T 5Y6

Volunteer Bureau
8 Albert Street East
Sault Ste. Marie, Ontario
P6A 2H6
(705) 949-6556

Volunteer Bureau of Leeds Grenville
187 King Street West
P.O. Box 1813
Brockville, Ontario
K6V 6K8
(613) 342-7040

Volunteer Centre of
Metropolitan Toronto
Etobicoke Branch
Burnhamthorpe Collegiate
Room 105
76 Keane Avenue
Etobicoke, Ontario
M9B 2C4
(417) 621-9936

Volunteer Centre of
Metropolitan Toronto
Scarborough Branch
Midland Avenue Collegiate
720 Midland Avenue
Scarborough, Ontario
M1K 4C9
(416) 264-2308

Volunteer Centre of Peel
Suite 705
30 Eglinton Avenue West
Mississauga, Ontario
L5R 3E7

Volunteer Services of
Windsor–Essex County
Unit F
1695 University Avenue West
Windsor, Ontario
N9B 1C3
(519) 253-6351

Volunteers Etobicoke
590 Rathburn Road
Etobicoke, Ontario
M9C 3T4
(416) 620-7837 or 620-7838

Walkerton & District Community
Support Services
Georgian Bay Council
P.O. Box #999
19 Durham Street East
Walkerton, Ontario
N0G 2V0
(519) 881-3713

Wallaceburg and Sydenham District
Association for Community Living
Lake St. Clair Council
939 Dufferin Avenue
Wallaceburg, Ontario
N8A 2V7
(519) 627-0776

Wawa & District Association for the
Mentally Retarded
Algoma Council
c/o Community Support Services
P.O. Box #193
Wawa, Ontario
P0S 1K0
(705) 856-2423

Welland District Association for
Community Living
Niagara Regional Council
30 East Main Street
Welland, Ontario
L3B 3W3
(416) 735-0081

West Nipissing Association for
Community Living
North Central Ontario Council
177 King Street
Box #1238
Sturgeon Falls, Ontario
P0H 2G0
(705) 753-1665

West Parry Sound Association for
Community Living
North Central Ontario Council
7 James Street
Parry Sound, Ontario
P2A 1T4
(705) 746-4254

Wikwemikong Anishinabe Association
for Community Living
Sudbury & Manitoulin Council
Wikwemikong, Ontario
P0P 2J0

Windsor Community Living
Support Services
Lake St. Clair Council
2090 Wyandotte Street East
Suite #201
Windsor, Ontario
N8Y 1E6
(519) 252-6751

Wingham and District Community
Living Association
Midwestern Ontario Council
P.O. Box #276
Wingham, Ontario
N0G 2W0
(519) 357-3562

Woodstock & District Developmental
Services
Midwestern Ontario Council
P.O. Box #188
Woodstock, Ontario
N4S 7W8
(519) 539-7447

York South Association for
Community Living
York Council
475 Edward Avenue
Richmond Hill, Ontario
L4C 5E5
(416) 884-9110

Ottawa and Vicinity

ADULT DAY CARE

Alzheimer "Day Away" Program
43 Bruyere Street
Ottawa, Ontario
234-4971

Alzheimer Day Away Program
Garde de Jour (Le Centre de Jour)
75 Bruyere Street
Ottawa, Ontario
234-4666
235-1847

Carleton Lodge
R.R. #2
Nepean, Ontario
825-3763

Centre d'accueil Champlain
275 Perrier Street
Vanier, Ontario
746-3543

The Good Companions Seniors Centre
670 Albert Street
Ottawa, Ontario
237-6879

Rothwell Heights Lodge
1735 Montreal Road
Ottawa, Ontario
744-2322

St. Patrick's Home
2865 Riverside Drive
Ottawa, Ontario
731-4660

ALERT SYSTEMS

Lifeline
560-1488

Medi-Call Canada
202 Catherine Street
Ottawa, Ontario
K2P 2K9
563-1935

Protectalert Information Centre
in Toronto
c/o Para-Med Health Services
1090 Ambleside Drive
Main Floor
Ottawa, Ontario
K2B 8G7
1-800-928-2666
820-3830

BEREAVEMENT SUPPORT

Bereaved Families of Ontario,
Ottawa–Carleton
P.O. Box 9384
Ottawa Terminal
Ottawa, Ontario
K1G 3V1
(613) 738-7171

Cumberland Township Home Support
1202 Colonial Road
Box 374
Navan, Ontario
K4B 1J5
(613) 835-3526

Gloucester Senior Adults' Centre
P.O. Box 8333
2020 Ogilvie Road
Gloucester, Ontario
K1G 3V5
(613) 749-1974

Gloucester Seniors
Coordinating Council
(613) 748-4130

Nepean Seniors Advisory Council
(613) 225-1973

Nepean Seniors' Home Support
Suite 245
Bell Mews Plaza
39 Robertson Road
Nepean, Ontario
K2H 8R2
(613) 829-1133

Ottawa–Carleton Regional Palliative
Care Association
(613) 560-1483

Rideau Seniors Advisory and
Referral Centre
P.O. Box 1218
Manotick, Ontario
K0A 2N0
(613) 692-2499

Township of Osgoode
Home Support Programme
c/o Township of Osgood Care Centre
R.R. #3
Metcalfe, Ontario
K0A 2P0
(613) 821-1978

Township of Rideau Senior Citizens
Centre Inc.
P.O. Box 423
Manotick Mews, John Street
Manotick, Ontario
K0A 2N0
(613) 692-4697

COMMUNITY AND SOCIAL SERVICES (COMSOC)

Government of Ontario
10 Rideau Street
Ottawa, Ontario
K1N 9J1
234-1188

Ottawa–Carleton Regional District
Health Council
955 Green Valley Crescent
Suite 350
Ottawa, Ontario
K2C 3V4
723-1440

Social Planning Council of
Ottawa–Carleton
256 King Edward Avenue
2nd Floor
Ottawa, Ontario
K1N 7M1
236-3658

CRISIS INTERVENTION SERVICES

Caring Hearts Homemaking Services
172 Rideau Street, Suite 2
Ottawa, Ontario
K1N 5X6
230-6140

Catholic Family Service of
Ottawa-Carlton
200 Isabella Street
4th Floor
Ottawa, Ontario
K1S 1V7
233-8478

Centre for Counselling and
Pastoral Service
Saint Paul University
223 Main Street
Ottawa, Ontario
236-1393

Centre for Psychological Services
University of Ottawa
6th Floor, Vanier Hall
275 Nicholas Street
Ottawa, Ontario
K1N 6N5
564-6875

Citizen Advocacy of Ottawa–Carleton
119 Ross Avenue
Suite 202
Ottawa, Ontario
K1Y 0N6
761-9522

Community Information Centre
260 St. Patrick Street
Ottawa, Ontario
K1N 5K5
238-2101

Concerned Friends, Ottawa
Paddy Bowen
28 Melgund Avenue
Ottawa, Ontario
K1S 2S2

Disabled Persons' Community
Resources
1525 Carling Avenue
Lower Level
Ottawa, Ontario
K1Z 8R9
724-5886

Family Service Centre of Ottawa
119 Ross Avenue
Ottawa, Ontario
K1Y 0N6
725-3601

Jewish Social Services Agency
151 Chapel Street
Ottawa, Ontario
K1N 7Y2
235-0000

Old Forge Community Resource Centre
2730 Carling Avenue
Ottawa, Ontario
K2B 7J1
829-9777

Ottawa Pastoral Centre
Anglican Diocese of Ottawa
439 Queen Street
Ottawa, Ontario
K1R 5A6
235-2516

Peer Counselling for Seniors
119 Ross Avenue
Ottawa, Ontario
K1Y 0N6
725-3601

Senior Citizens Council of
Ottawa–Carleton Inc.
294 Albert Street
Room 508
Ottawa, Ontario
K1P 6E6
234-8044

Widowed Support Group of
Ottawa–Carleton
P.O. Box 16087
Station F
Ottawa, Ontario
K2C 3S9
738-3374

DAY CARE HOSPITALS

Geriatric Day Care Hospital
75 Bruyere Street
4th Floor
Ottawa, Ontario
560-1471

Match and Share Seniors Home
Sharing Program
222 Queen Street
10th Floor
Ottawa, Ontario
K1P 5Z3
560-1366

Queensway-Carleton Hospital
3045 Baseline Road
Nepean, Ontario
721-2000

Royal Ottawa Hospital
1145 Carling Avenue
Ottawa, Ontario
722-6521

St. Vincent Hospital
60 Cambridge Street, North
Ottawa, Ontario
233-4041

DAY CENTRES AND DROP-IN CENTRES

Abbotsford House Seniors Centre
954 Bank Street
Ottawa, Ontario
K1S 5G6
230-5730

Adults For Lively Leisure (A.L.L.)
235-0000

Le Centre de jour Polyvalent des Aines
Francophones d'Ottawa–Carleton
75 Bruyere Street
1st Floor
Ottawa, Ontario
K1N 5C7
235-1847

Churchill Senior Citizens
Drop-In Centre
345 Richmond Road
Ottawa, Ontario
K2A 0E7
564-1016

Good Companions Seniors Centre
670 Albert Street
Ottawa, Ontario
K1R 6L2
236-0428

The Italo-Canadian Senior
Citizens Group
10 Balsam Street
Ottawa, Ontario
233-9298

Jack Purcell Community Centre
320 Elgin Street
Ottawa, Ontario
K2P 2J5
564-1050

Jewish Community Centre
151 Chapel Street
Ottawa, Ontario
K1N 7Y2
232-7306

Kiwanian Alex Dayton Senior
Activity Centre
728-5341

Le Patro d'Ottawa
Le Club de l'amitie
40 Cobourg Street
Ottawa, Ontario
K1N 8Z6
233-7733

RA Seniors Club
c/o RA Centre
2451 Riverside Drive
Ottawa, Ontario
K1H 7X7
733-5100

Seniors' Resource Centre
University of Ottawa
192 Laurier Avenue East
Ottawa, Ontario
K1N 6N5
564-2941
564-2972

South East Ottawa Community
Resource Centre
1480 Heron Road
Ottawa, Ontario
K1V 6A5
737-5115

South-East Ottawa Senior
Action Group
1480 Heron Road
Ottawa, Ontario
K1V 6A5
738-1224

Yet Keen Day Centre
80 Florence Street
Ottawa, Ontario
K1R 5N2
232-8403

FRIENDLY VISITING

The Good Companions Seniors
Reach Out (Wednesday and Friday)
237-6879

Italo Canadian Senior Citizens Group
233-9298

Jewish Social Services Agency
235-0000

Olde Forge Seniors Support Service
737-5115

Ottawa West Seniors' Support
728-6016

Seniors Outreach Services,
Glebe Centre
230-5730

Service d'Entraide communautaire
237-1266

HOME SUPPORT SERVICE AGENCIES

Abbotsford House Seniors Centre
230-5730

Churchill Senior Citizens Centre
564-1016

Glebe Centre Inc.
Luncheon Club Program
950 Bank Street
Ottawa, Ontario
K1S 5G6
230-5730

Good Companion Wheels to Meals
670 Albert Street
Ottawa, Ontario
K1R 6L2
236-0428

Good Companions Seniors Centre
670 Albert Street
Ottawa, Ontario
K1R 6L2
237-6879

Grocery Express
70 Spencer Street
Ottawa, Ontario
K1Y 4P1
725-1222

Home Support Services
Social Services Department
Regional Municipality of
Ottawa–Carleton
330 Lajoie Street
Vanier, Ontario
K1L 7H4
744-2892

Jewish Social Services Agency
151 Chapel Street
Ottawa, Ontario
K1N 7Y2
235-0000

Old Forge Seniors Support Service
2730 Carling Avenue
Ottawa, Ontario
K2B 7J1
829-9777

Ottawa West Seniors' Support
1137 Wellington Street
Ottawa, Ontario
K1Y 2Y8
728-6016

Para-Med Health Services
1090 Ambleside Drive
Suite 101
Ottawa, Ontario
K2B 8G7
820-3830

RA Seniors Club
733-5100

Seniors' Outreach Services (S.O.S.)
(Abbotsford House Seniors Centre)
954 Bank Street
Ottawa, Ontario
K1S 5G6
230-5730

Service d'Entraide communautaire
75 Bruyer Street
2nd Floor
Ottawa, Ontario
K1N 5C7
237-1266

South-East Ottawa Community
Resource Centre
1480 Heron Road
Ottawa, Ontario
K1V 6A5
737-5115

Visiting Homemakers Association
of Ottawa
880 Wellington Street
Suite 204
City Centre Bldg.
Ottawa, Ontario
728-2550

HOME SUPPORT SERVICES

Home Care Program (Acute Care and
Chronic Care)
Ottawa–Carleton Health Department
1223 Michael Street
4th Floor
Gloucester, Ontario
K1J 7T2
745-5525

Integrated Homemaker Program
722-2029

HUMAN AND CIVIL RIGHTS

Ombudsman of Ontario
Regional Office
151 Slater Street
Suite 702
Ottawa, Ontario
K1P 5H3
234-6421

LEISURE TIME ACTIVITIES

Home Reader Service
598-4017

Yiddish Mobile Library (JSSA)
235-0000

MEDICAL ASSESSMENT: GERIATRIC ASSESSMENT PROGRAM

Ottawa Civic Hospital
1053 Carling Avenue
Ottawa, Ontario
K1Y 4E9
761-4485

Ottawa General Hospital
501 Smyth Road
Ottawa, Ontario
K1H 8L6
737-7777

NURSING SERVICES

Community Nursing Registry
130 Somerset Street West
Suite 804
Ottawa, Ontario
K2P 0H9
236-3639

Public Health Nursing Division
Ottawa–Carleton Health Department
495 Richmond Road
Ottawa, Ontario
K2A 4A4
722-2242

Victorian Order of Nurses
5335 Canotek Road
Gloucester, Ontario
K1J 9L4
749-7557

OTHER FORMS OF ASSISTANCE

Anglican Social Service Centre
454 King Edward Avenue
Ottawa, Ontario
K1N 7M8
235-4351
235-4352

Canadian Red Cross Society
(Ottawa–Carleton)
85 Plymouth Street
Ottawa, Ontario
K1S 3E2
560-7440

Good Companions—Income Tax
Counselling Service
670 Albert Street
Ottawa, Ontario
K1R 6L2
236-0428

Ottawa Carleton Health Department
495 Richmond Road
Ottawa, Ontario
K2A 4A4
722-2242
745-5525
564-1111

Ottawa West Seniors' Support
1137 Wellington Street
Ottawa, Ontario
K1Y 2Y8
728-6016

PLANNING AND COORDINATION AGENCIES

The Council on Aging
Social Planning Council of
Ottawa–Carleton
256 King Edward Avenue
Ottawa, Ontario
K1N 7M1
232-3577

REASSURANCE

Letter Carriers' Alert Program
Senior Citizens Council of
Ottawa–Carleton Inc.
294 Albert Street
Room 508
Ottawa, Ontario
K1P 6E6
234-8044

Telephone Assurance Program (TAP)
Community Information Centre
260 St. Patrick Street
Suite 301
Ottawa, Ontario
K1N 5K5
238-2101

Teleshalom (Jewish Social Services)
235-0000

SELF-HELP GROUPS

Alzheimer Society of Ottawa–Carleton
1525 Carling Avenue, Lower Level
Ottawa, Ontario
K1Z 8R9

At Home-Chez Nous
c/o Elsa Zilberbogen
150 MacLaren, #305
Ottawa, Ontario
K2P 0L2

Canadian Hearing Society
Ottawa & District Regional Office
216 Murray Street
Ottawa, Ontario
K1N 5N1
236-0509
236-0902

Canadian National Institute
for the Blind
320 McLeod Street
Ottawa, Ontario
K2P 1A3
563-4021

Centre Volunteer Bureau of
Ottawa–Carleton
256 King Edward Avenue
Ottawa, Ontario
K1N 7M1
232-4876

Council on Aging of Ottawa–Carleton
256 King Edward Avenue
Ottawa, Ontario
K1N 7M1
232-3577

Heart and Stroke Foundation of Canada
Suite 200
160 George Street
Ottawa, Ontario
K1N 9M2
237-4361

National Voluntary Organizations
P.O. Box 15812, Station F
Ottawa, Ontario
K2C 3S7

The Old Forge
Community Resource Centre
2730 Carling Avenue
Ottawa, Ontario
K2B 7J1
829-9777

Ottawa and District Association for the
Mentally Retarded
Champlain Council
55 Parkdale Avenue North
3rd floor
Ottawa, Ontario
K1Y 1E5

Placement Co-ordination Service of
Ottawa–Carleton
955 Green Valley Crescent, Room 380
Ottawa, Ontario
K2C 3V4

Senior Citizens Council of
Ottawa–Carleton
294 Albert Street, Room 508
Ottawa, Ontario
K1Z 8R9

Seniors Guide to Federal Services
& Programs
Seniors
P.O. Box 8176
Ottawa, Ontario
K1G 3H7

SENIOR CITIZENS ASSOCIATIONS

Federation of Francophone
Senior Citizens of Ontario
75 Bruyere Street
Room 3738
J Wing
Ottawa, Ontario
K1N 5C7
235-4258

National Advisory Council on Aging
Room 340, Brooke Claxton Building
Tunney's Pasture
Ottawa, Ontario
K1A 0K6

One Voice Seniors Network
(Canada) Inc.
350 Sparks Street
Suite 901
Ottawa, Ontario
K1R 7S8
238-7624

SENIORS ORGANIZATIONS

The Francophone Association of Senior
Citizens of Ottawa–Carleton
75 Bruyere Street
Ottawa, Ontario
K1N 5C7
235-3952

Senior Citizens Council of
Ottawa–Carleton, Inc.
294 Albert Street
Room 508
Ottawa, Ontario
K1P 6E6
234-8044

SICK ROOM EQUIPMENT

Alzheimer Day Away Program
75 Bruyere Street
Ottawa, Ontario
K1N 5C8
234-4971

Alzheimer and Related Disorders Unit
Psycho-Geriatric Clinic
232 Cumberland Street
Ottawa, Ontario
K1N 7H5
234-4666

Alzheimer Society
1525 Carling Avenue
Lower Level
Ottawa, Ontario
K1Z 8R9
722-1424

The Arthritis Society
1129 Carling Avenue
Ottawa, Ontario
K1Y 4G8
728-2685

Canadian Cancer Society
200 Melrose Avenue
Ottawa, Ontario
K1Y 4K7
722-7635

Canadian Red Cross Society
85 Plymouth Street
Ottawa, Ontario
K1N 3E2
560-7440

Heart and Stroke Foundation of Canada
160 George Street
Room 200
Ottawa, Ontario
K1N 4M2
237-4361

Heart and Stroke Foundation
of Ontario
(Ottawa–Carleton Chapter)
1729 Bank Street
Room 303
Ottawa, Ontario
K1V 7Z5
733-2096

Kidney Foundation, Ottawa Chapter
212-1335 Carling Avenue
Ottawa, Ontario
K1Z 8N8
724-9953

Multiple Sclerosis Society of Canada
510-880 Wellington Street
Ottawa, Ontario
K1R 6K7
232-4278

Osteoporosis Information Centre
OSTOP Ottawa
220-1320 Richmond Road
Ottawa, Ontario
K2B 8L3
596-9374

Ottawa Stroke Association
P.O. Box 5550
Station F
Ottawa, Ontario
K2C 3M1
526-3549

Parkinson's Disease Society of
Ottawa–Carleton
Ottawa Civic Hospital
1053 Carling Avenue
Ottawa, Ontario
K1Y 4E9
722-9368

Toronto and Vicinity

CANADIAN CANCER SOCIETY— NEIGHBOURHOOD UNITS

Agincourt Unit
70 Silver Star Blvd.
Unit 114
Scarborough, Ontario
M1V 4V9
293-7422

Beaches Riverdale Unit
1958 Gerrard Street East
Toronto, Ontario
M4E 2B2
691-9454

Central Toronto Unit
20 Holly Street
Suite 101
Toronto, Ontario
M4B 1B1
485-0222

Don Mills Unit
1262 Don Mills Road
#66
Don Mills, Ontario
M3B 2W7
447-6120

Downsview Unit
356 Wilson Avenue
Downsview, Ontario
M3H 1S9
636-0421

East York Unit
470 Mortimer Avenue
#105
Toronto, Ontario
M4J 2G5
465-9203

Etobicoke Unit
4920 Dundas Street West
Suite 306
Box 292, Station D
Etobicoke, Ontario
M9A 4X2
231-1118

Humber/Keele Unit
159 Jane Street
Toronto, Ontario
M6S 3Y8
762-5749

Rexdale Unit
988 Albion Road
Rexdale, Ontario
M9V 1A7
741-4062

Scarborough Unit
3750 St. Clair Avenue East
Scarborough, Ontario
M1M 1T9
261-6942

West Hill Unit
4512 Kingston Road
Scarborough, Ontario
M1E 2N8
283-7023

West Toronto Unit
1011 Dufferin Street
Suite 202
Toronto, Ontario
M6H 4B5
532-3318

Weston Unit
1901 Weston Road
Unit 6
Weston, Ontario
247-3664

Willowdale Unit
6075 Yonge Street
4th Floor
Willowdale, Ontario
M2M 3W2
226-0646

HOME CARE PROGRAMS

Canadian Cancer Society
Patient Services
2 Carlton Street
Toronto, Ontario
M5B 2J2
593-1513

Care Ring for Rexdale
925 Albion Road
Rexdale, Ontario
M9V 1A6
745-4472

Central Neighbourhood House
Home Support
264 Seaton Street #100
Toronto, Ontario
M5A 2TA
966-8595

Comcare Ltd.
Homecare
15 Madison Avenue
Toronto, Ontario
929-3364

Community Care East York
Respite Care Program
334 Donlands Avenue
Toronto, Ontario
M4J 3R9
422-2026

Downsview Services to Seniors
Caregiver Relief Service
15 Clubhouse Ct.
Downsview, Ontario
M3L 2L7
633-9519

Etobicoke Red Cross
Homemaker Service
4210 Dundas Street West
Etobicoke, Ontario
M8X 1Y6
236-1791

Greek Community of Metropolitan
Toronto Inc.
Home Support Services
759 Pape Avenue
Toronto, Ontario
M4K 3T2
469-1155

Kimberly Quality Care
720 Spadina Avenue, Suite 402
Toronto, Ontario
922-3244

Medcare/Personicare Partnership
Homecare Program
1992 Yonge Street, #306
Toronto, Ontario
M4S 12Z
484-4433

Parkdale Golden Age Foundation
Friendly Visiting, In-home
1605 Queen Street West
Toronto, Ontario
M6R 1A9
536-6077

Scarborough Support Services for the
Elderly Inc.
Scarborough In-Home Respite Program
425 McCowan Road
Scarborough, Ontario
M1J 1J1
439-5012

Selectacare
139 Sheppard Avenue East
Willowdale, Ontario
M2N 3A6
225-8900

Senior Care
Respite Care Program
530 Wilson Avenue, 3rd Floor
North York, Ontario
M3H 1T6
635-2860

Senior Link
Home Support
2550 Danforth Avenue
Toronto, Ontario
M4C 1L2
489-2500

Senior People's Resources in North
Toronto (Sprint)
Respite Care Program
641 Eglinton Avenue West
Toronto, Ontario
M5N 1C5
481-6411

Seniors for Seniors
55 Eglinton Avenue East
#803
Toronto, Ontario
M4P 1G8
481-2733

St. Paul's L'Amoreaux Centre
Scarborough In-Home Respite Program
3333 Finch Avenue East
Scarborough, Ontario
M1W 2R9
493-3333

Upjohn Health Care Services
Home Support, Caregiver Relief
156 Front Street West, #304
Toronto, Ontario
M5J 2L6

York Community Services
York Co-ordinated Respite Program
1651 Keele Street
Toronto, Ontario
M6M 3W2
653-5400

SELF-HELP CLEARING HOUSES

Self Help Clearing House of
Metro Toronto
215-40 Orchard View Blvd.
Toronto, Ontario
M4R 1B9
487-4355

SELF-HELP GROUPS

Advocacy Centre for the Elderly
Toronto, Ontario
487-7157

Alzheimer Association of Ontario
Suite 423
131 Bloor Street West
Toronto, Ontario
M5S 1R1
967-5900

Bereaved Families of Ontario
Toronto, Ontario
440-0290

Bloor Information and Legal Services
1072 Dovercourt Road
Toronto, Ontario
M6H 2X8
531-4613

Canadian Cystic Fibrosis Foundation
Suite 601
2221 Yonge Street
Toronto, Ontario
M4S 2B4
485-9149

City of Toronto Information Services
Toronto, Ontario
392-7341/TDD 392-7354

Community Information
for the City of York
2696 Eglinton Avenue West
York, Ontario
M6M 1T9
652-2273

Community Information Centre of
Metropolitan Toronto
590 Jarvis Street
5th floor
Toronto, Ontario
M4Y 2J4
392-0505

Community Information Fairview
Fairview Mall, Box U219A
1800 Sheppard Avenue East
North York, Ontario
M2J 5A7
493-0752

Connect Information Post
1589 Dupont Street, 2nd floor
Toronto, Ontario
M6P 3S5
534-3561

Dial-a-Law
Toronto, Ontario
947-3333

Elder Abuse
Community Information Centre
Toronto, Ontario
392-0505

Elder Abuse
Downtown Health Area
City of Toronto Department of
Public Health
Toronto, Ontario
392-7462

Elder Abuse
Eastern Health Area
City of Toronto Department of
Public Health
Toronto, Ontario
392-0936

Elder Abuse
Metro Police
Toronto, Ontario
324-2222

Elder Abuse
Northern Health Area
City of Toronto Department of
Public Health
Toronto, Ontario
392-0962

Elder Abuse
Western Health Area
City of Toronto Department of
Public Health
Toronto, Ontario
392-0983

Emergency Shelter
Metro Homes for the Aged
Toronto, Ontario
392-8928/after hours 392-0505

Extended Care Program
Public Enquiry Centre
Ontario Ministry of Health
50 Grosvenor Street
Toronto, Ontario
965-1506

Financial Assistance
Metro Community Services
Toronto, Ontario
598-1121/486-1456

Fitness & Recreation
City of Toronto Department of
Parks and Recreation
Toronto, Ontario
392-7259

GO Transit
Toronto, Ontario

Health Information
Downtown Health Area
City of Toronto Department of
Public Health
Toronto, Ontario
392-7426

Health Information
Eastern Health Area
City of Toronto Department of
Public Health
Toronto, Ontario
392-0936

Health Information
Northern Health Area
City of Toronto Department of
Public Health
Toronto, Ontario
392-0962

Health Information
Western Health Area
City of Toronto Department of
Public Health
Toronto, Ontario
392-0983

Health Information
Ontario Ministry of Health
Toronto, Ontario
965-3101

Heart and Stroke Foundation
of Ontario
4th Floor
477 Mount Pleasant Road
Toronto, Ontario
M4S 2L9
489-7100

Home Care Program for
Metropolitan Toronto
Toronto, Ontario
229-2929

Home Renewal Programs
City of Toronto Housing Department
Toronto, Ontario
392-7620

Home Support Services
Community Information Centre
Toronto, Ontario
392-0505

Home Support Services
Seniors Information Centre
Toronto, Ontario
965-5103

Information Downsview
Brookview Middle School
4505 Jane Street
Downsview, Ontario
M3N 2K7
633-1067 (Info)
736-9467 (Admin)

Information for Seniors
Community Information Centre of
Metropolitan Toronto
Toronto, Ontario
392-0505

Information Scarborough
4139 Sheppard Avenue East
Scarborough, Ontario
M1S 1T1
321-6912

Landlords Self Help Centre
Toronto, Ontario
532-4467

Lawyer Referral Service
Toronto, Ontario
947-3330

Legal Services
Community Information Centre
Toronto, Ontario
392-0505

LINK Community Information and
Referral Centre
North York Public Library
5120 Yonge Street
North York, Ontario
M2N 5N9
395-5591
295-5596 (TDD)

Metro Homes for the Aged
Toronto, Ontario
392-8928

Metro Tenants Legal Services
Toronto, Ontario
926-9693

Metropolitan Toronto Association for
Community Living
Metropolitan Toronto Council
20 Spadina Road
Toronto, Ontario
M5R 2S7
968-0650

Metropolitan Toronto Convention &
Visitors Association
Toronto, Ontario
368-9821

Metropolitan Toronto Reference
Library
Toronto, Ontario
393-7131

The Multiple Sclerosis Society
of Canada
National Office
Suite 820
250 Bloor Street East
Toronto, Ontario
M4W 3P9
922-6065

The Multiple Sclerosis Society
of Canada
Ontario Division
Suite 820
250 Bloor Street East
Toronto, Ontario
M4W 3P9
922-6065

Neighbourhood Information Centre
91 Barrington Avenue
Toronto, Ontario
M4C 4Y9
698-1626

Neighbourhood Information Post
265 Gerrard Street East
Toronto, Ontario
M5A 2G3
924-2543

Nutrition and Food
City of Toronto Department of
Public Health
Toronto, Ontario
392-7451

Nutrition and Food
Ontario Ministry of
Agriculture & Food
Toronto, Ontario
326-3418

Ontario Legal Aid
Toronto, Ontario
598-0200

Ontario Office for Senior Citizens
(Guide for Senior Citizens)
Toronto, Ontario
965-5106

Parkdale Community
Information Centre
1303 Queen Street West
Toronto, Ontario
M6K 1L6
392-7689

Parkinson Foundation of Canada
Suite 232
55 Bloor Street West
Toronto, Ontario
M4W 1A5
964-1155

Reference Canada
Toronto, Ontario
973-1993

Rent Review Services
Ontario Ministry of Housing
Toronto, Ontario
964-8281

Retirement Plus
Volunteer Centre of
Metropolitan Toronto
Toronto, Ontario
961-6888

Seniors Central Housing Registry
Toronto, Ontario
392-6111

Seniors Centres & Clubs
Community Information Centre
Toronto, Ontario
392-0505

Seniors Information Service
Toronto, Ontario
965-5103

Snow Clearing
City of Toronto Department of
Public Works
Toronto, Ontario
392-7768

Toronto Mayor's Committee on Aging
Newsletter
Toronto, Ontario
392-0129 (answering machine)

Toronto Transit Commission
Toronto, Ontario

Travelling Library
Toronto Public Libraries
Toronto, Ontario
393-7644

TTC Card
Metro Community Services
Toronto, Ontario
398-8701

Via Rail
Toronto, Ontario

Volunteer Centre of
Metropolitan Toronto
344 Bloor Street West
Suite 207
Toronto, Ontario
M5S 1W9
961-6888

Volunteer Centre of
Metropolitan Toronto
East York Branch
Community Care East York
334 Donlands Avenue
Toronto, Ontario
M4J 3R9
467-1327

Volunteer Centre of
Metropolitan Toronto
North York Branch
Armour Heights Public School
148 Wilson Avenue
Toronto, Ontario
M5M 3A5
264-2308

Volunteer Centre of
Metropolitan Toronto
York Branch
Rawlinson Community School
Room 207C
231 Glenholme Avenue
Toronto, Ontario
M6E 3C7
658-6160

SENIOR CITIZENS ASSOCIATIONS

Canadian Association of
Retired Persons
27 Queen Street East
Suite 304
Toronto, Ontario
M5C 2M6
363-8748

Canadian Council of Retirees
c/o Canadian Labour Congress
15 Gervais Drive
Room 305
Don Mills, Ontario
M3C 1Y8
441-3710

Canadian Pensioners Concerned
51 Bond Street
Toronto, Ontario
M5B 1X1
368-5222

Home Support Association of Ontario
c/o Mr. Paul Tuttle, President
Durham Region Community Care
Association
P.O. Box 300
Dundas Street West
Whitby, Ontario
L1N 5S3
668-6583

Mrs. Dorothea Knights
1412 Parent Avenue
Windsor, Ontario
N8X 4J5

Meals on Wheels of Ontario Inc.
43 Eglinton Avenue East
Suite 804
Toronto, Ontario
M4P 1A2
489-2195

National Pensioners and Senior
Citizens' Federation
3033 Lakeshore Boulevard West
Toronto, Ontario
M8V 1K5
251-7042

Older Adults Centres Association
of Ontario
1220 Sheppard Avenue, East
Suite 409
Willowdale, Ontario
M2X 2X1
495-4061

Ontario Advisory Council on
Senior Citizens
700 Bay Street
Suite 203
Toronto, Ontario
M5G 1Z6
965-2324

Ontario Association of
Non-Profit Homes
and Services for Seniors (OANHSS)
7 Director Court, Suite 102
Woodbridge, Ontario
L4L 4S5
851-8821

United Senior Citizens of Ontario
3033 Lakeshore Boulevard West
Toronto, Ontario
M8V 1K5
252-2021

QUEBEC

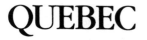

ASSOCIATION CANADIENNE POUR LA SANTE MENTALE

Filiani de Chicoutimi
C P 951
Chicoutimi, Quebec
G7H 5E8

Mme. Gisele Duguay
ACSM—Filiale de Gaspe
C P 126
Gaspe, Quebec
G0C 1R0

Mme. Johanne Blais
Directrice
Association Canadienne pour
la Sante Mentale
Filiale de l'Outaouais
672, boul. St-Joseph
Hull, Quebec
J8Y 4A8

M. Jacques Duval
Directeur
Association Canadienne pour
la Sante Mentale
Filiale de Montreal
874, rue Cherrier
#201
Montreal, Quebec
H2L 1H6

Mme. Christine Berryman
Directrice
Association Canadienne pour
la Sante Mentale
Filiale de Quebec
432, boul. St-Cyrille Ouest
Quebec, P.Q.
G1S 1S3

Mme. Alice Berge
Association Canadianne pour
la Sante Mentale
Filiale Bas-du-Bleuve
C P 593
Rimouski, Quebec
G5L 4X7

Filiale du Lac St-Jean
C P 131
680, boul. St-Joseph
#208
Robervale, Quebec
G8H 2N6

Filiale de Sherbrooke
72, rue Victoria
Sherbrooke, Quebec
J1H 3H7

Filiale de Sorel
189, rue Prince
#311
Sorel, Quebec
J3P 4K6

M. Dominique Gagnon
ACSM—Filiale de Valleyfield
55, rue Madeleine
Valleyfield, Quebec
J6S 3S3

CANADIAN ASSOCIATION FOR COMMUNITY LIVING

Quebec Association for
Community Living
3440, avenue de l'hotel-de-ville
Montreal, Quebec
H2X 3B4
(514) 849-3616

FAMILY SERVICE CANADA

Centre de services sociaux de
Montreal metropolitain
1001, boul. de Maisonneuve est
Montreal, Quebec
H2L 4R5
(514) 527-7261

C.L.S.C. St-Leonard
6025 Jean-Talon est, Suite 210
St-Leonard, Quebec
H1S 1M6
(514) 252-1030

Confederation des organismes
familiaux du Quebec
4098 rue St-Hubert
Montreal, Quebec
H2L 4A8
(514) 521-4777

Consultation-Familles Enr.
R.R. #6
Coaticook, Quebec
J1A 2S5
(819) 849-4278

Service de Promotion Famille
740 boul. Ste-Foy, C.P. 40
Longueuil, Quebec
J4K 4X8
(514) 679-1100

OCCUPATIONAL THERAPISTS

La corporation professionelle des
ergotherapeutes du Quebec (CPEQ)
1259, rue Berri, Suite 710
Montreal, Quebec
H2L 4C7
(514) 844-5778

THE PARKINSON FOUNDATION OF CANADA

Montreal, Quebec
(514) 866-2511

Pointe Claire, Quebec
(514) 630-2939

RED CROSS

Canadian Red Cross Society
Quebec
2170 Rene Levesque Blvd. West
Montreal, Quebec
H3H 1R6

SELF-HELP CLEARING HOUSES

Camac, Centre D'Aide Mutuelle
C.P. 535, Succ. Desjardins
Montreal, P.Q.
H5B 1B6
(514) 484-7406

SELF-HELP GROUPS

American Association of Marriage &
Family Therapists
c/o Montreal Family Institute
904 Avenue Dunlop
Outremont, Quebec
H2V 2W8
(514) 733-0124/737-2103

Federation des Centres D'Action
Benevole du Quebec
928 St. Joseph Est
Montreal, Quebec
H2J 1K6
(514) 524-7515

La Federation Quebecoise des
Societes Alzheimer
1474 Fleury Est
Montreal, Quebec
H2C 1S1
(514) 388-3148

Heart and Stroke Foundation
of Quebec
Suite 1400
440 Rene-Levesque Boulevard West
Montreal, Quebec
H2Z 1V7
(514) 871-1551

The Multiple Sclerosis Society
of Canada
Quebec Division
Suite 401
279 Sherbrooke Street West
Montreal, Quebec
H2X 1Y2
(514) 849-7591

Volunteer Bureau of Montreal
1246 rue Bishop
Montreal, Quebec
H3G 2E3
(514) 866-3351

NOVA SCOTIA

ADULT SERVICE CENTRES

Anchor Industries
Sackville Industrial Park
61 Glendale Avenue
Lower Sackville, Nova Scotia
B4C 3J7
Manager: Cathy Deagle
865-1651

The Ark Industries
R. R. #1
Bridgewater, Nova Scotia
B4V 2V9
Manager: Cheryl Cooper
543-5308

Atelier de Clare
Universite Sainte-Anne
Church Point
Digby, Nova Scotia
B0W 1M0
Manager: Helen Lewis
769-3202

Beehive Adult Service Centre
Commercial Street
Aylesford, Kings Co., Nova Scotia
B0P 1C0
Manager: Carol Craig
847-9443

Brass Tack Workshop
40 MacLean Street
Glace Bay, Nova Scotia
B1A 2K7
Manager: Shirley Romo

The Bridge Adult Service Centre
10 Croft Street
Amherst, Nova Scotia
B4H 2Z4
Manager: Ms. Susan Thibodeau
667-8433

CAMR Community Workshop
83 Saint Ninian Street
Box 1330
Antigonish Co., Nova Scotia
B2G 1Y7
Manager: Mr. Leonard MacDonald
863-5024

Colchester Community Workshops
575 Prince Street
Truro, Nova Scotia
B2N 1G2
Manager: Ann Cooper
893-7228

The Conway Workshop
R.R. #2
Digby, Nova Scotia
B0V 1A0
Manager: Troy Guindon
245-5391

DASC Industries
10 Akerley Blvd.
Suite 24
Burnside Industrial Park
Dartmouth, Nova Scotia
B3B 1J4
Manager: Sandra Purcell
469-0856

Endale Industries
P.O. Box 251
Elmsdale, Nova Scotia
B0N 1M0
Manager: Linda Horne
883-9404

The Flower Cart
1196 Commercial Street
New Minas, Nova Scotia
B4N 3E9
Manager: Jim Oulton
678-2478

Golden Opportunity Vocational and
Rehabilitation Centre
25 King Street
Springhill, Nova Scotia
B0M 1X0
Manager: Mrs. Joanne Hunter
597-3158

The Green Door Society Ltd.
P.O. Box 366
Cheticamp, Nova Scotia
B0E 1H0
Manager: Georgina Poirier
224-2000

Halifax Adult Service Centre
3430 Prescott Street
Halifax, Nova Scotia
B3K 4Y4
Manager: Susan Slaunwhite
454-7387

Heatherton Adult Service Centre
P.O. Box 35
Heatherton, Antigonish Co.,
Nova Scotia
B0H 1R0
Manager: Ms. Jovita Chisholm
386-2808

Kay Nickerson Adult Service Centre
83 Parade Street
Yarmouth, Nova Scotia
B5A 4B1
Manager: Hubert Devine
742-2238

Northside Adult Service Centre
26 Haley Street
North Sydney, Nova Scotia
Manager: Debra MacLean
794-3517

Queens Adult Service Centre
P.O. Box 100
Liverpool, Nova Scotia
B0T 1K0
Manager: Murray Kirkpatrick
354-2723

Regional Occupational Centre
Vocational School Residence
P.O. Box 839
Port Hawkesbury, Nova Scotia
B0E 2V0
Manager: Kay Isenor
625-0132

Revolving Door
Annapolis East CAMR
P.O. Box 45
Lawrencetown, Nova Scotia
B0S 1M0
Chairperson: Tom Porter
584-3332

Shelburne County Adult Mentally
Handicapped Workshop
P.O. Box 356
Barrington Passage, Nova Scotia
B0W 1G0
Manager: Marion Boudreau
875-2668

Summer Street Industries
874 Summer Street
New Glasgow, Nova Scotia
B2H 3Z2
Manager: Bob Bennett
755-1945

Sydney Kinsmen Resource Centre
780 Prince Street
Sydney, Nova Scotia
B1P 5N6
Manager: Mary Lynne O'Leary
539-8553

Windsor Adult Vocational
Services Centre
P.O. Box 1075
6 Centennial Drive
Windsor, Nova Scotia
B0N 2T0
Manager: Dorothy Miller-Fleet
798-5160

CANADIAN ASSOCIATION FOR COMMUNITY LIVING

Canadian Association for Community
Living—Nova Scotia Division
83 Portland Street
Dartmouth, Nova Scotia
B2Y 1H5
469-1174

CANADIAN MENTAL HEALTH ASSOCIATION

Ms. Anne Forbes
CMHA—Dartmouth Branch
152 Prince Albert Road
Dartmouth, Nova Scotia
B2Y 1M5

Mrs. Irene Drake Smith
Administrative Director
CMHA—Halifax Branch
5739 Inglis Street
Halifax, Nova Scotia
B3H 1K5

Ms. Barbara McKinnon
Program & Information Officer
CMHA—Cape Breton Branch
P.O. Box 515
Sydney, Nova Scotia
B1P 6H4

COORDINATED HOME CARE

Antigonish & Area Homemaker Service
863-6477

Town of Canso Homemaker Services
366-3488

Cape Breton County Homemaker
Agency, 562-5003

Children's Aid & Family Services of
Colchester Co., 893-5950
893-0500

Family & Children's Services of
Cumberland County, 667-0870

City of Dartmouth, 464-2380

Digby Area, 245-5811

Dominion Visiting Homemaker Service
849-1202

Citizens Service League of Glace Bay
849-3252

Guysborough County Homemaker
Services, 533-3655

City of Halifax
Halifax Community Care—Home Care
421-6407
421-2747

Municipality of Halifax County
Homemakers Services
864-1147
864-1146

Homemakers Services of Hants County
798-4452

Inverness County Homemaker Services
787-2714

Kings County Homemaker Services
678-6141

Family & Children's Services of
Lunenburg County
543-2411
543-1167

Town of Mulgrave Homemakers
Services, 747-2243

New Waterford Homemaker Service
Society, 862-7554

Northside Visiting Homemaker Service
Society, 736-2701

Pictou County Visiting Homemakers
752-0560

Town of Port Hawkesbury Homemaker
Services, 625-2746

Queens County Homemakers
354-2771
354-3333

Richmond County Homemaker Services
535-2828

Shelburne Area, 637-3588

St. Mary's Homemaker Service Society
522-2861

City Homemakers Service Society
Sydney, 564-0460

Victoria County Homemaker Service
295-2764

Town of Wolfville Homemaker Services
542-5767

Yarmouth Area, 742-0906

FAMILY SERVICE CANADA

Family Service Association of Halifax,
Dartmouth, Bedford, Halifax County
5614 Fenwick Street
Halifax, Nova Scotia
B3H 1P9
420-1980

Family Service of Eastern Nova Scotia
69 King's Road
Sydney, Nova Scotia
B1S 1A2
539-0620

MUNICIPAL SOCIAL SERVICE WORKERS

Rosemary Mullins
Director of Social Services
P.O. Box 399
24 Crescent Avenue
Amherst, Nova Scotia
B4H 3Z5

Beverly McQuarrie
Director of Social Services
P.O. Box 471
Amherst, Nova Scotia
B4H 4A1

Brian Taylor
Director of Social Services
Municipal Administration Building
P.O. Box 100
Annapolis Royal, Nova Scotia
B0S 1P0

L.A. Mills
District Supervisor
Antigonish District Office
Suite 101
11 James Street
Antigonish, Nova Scotia
B2G 1R6

Ed Mason
Director of Social Services
P.O. Box 300
Armdale, Nova Scotia
B3L 4K3

Raymond G. Harris
District Supervisor
Shelburne District Office
P.O. Box 9
Barrington, Nova Scotia
B0W 1E0

James Kenny
Acting District Supervisor
Lunenburg District Office
Suite 105
99 High Street
Bridgewater, Nova Scotia
B4V 1V8

Paul Greene
Director of Social Services
P.O. Box 817
Dartmouth, Nova Scotia
B2Y 3Z3

Greg Wiseman
District Supervisor
Digby District Office
P.O. Box 399
Digby, Nova Scotia
B0V 1A0

Greg MacKenzie
Director of Social Services
271 Kings Road
Dominion, Nova Scotia
B0A 1E0

Greg MacKenzie
Director of Social Services
R.R. #1
Glace Bay, Nova Scotia
B1A 5T9

Harold M. Roberts
District Supervisor
P.O. Box 90
Guysborough, Nova Scotia
B0H 1N0

Harold Crowell
Social Planner
City of Halifax
P.O. Box 1749
Halifax, Nova Scotia
B3K 3A5

Henry Bourgeois
Director of Social Services
P.O. Box 100
Kentville, Nova Scotia
B4N 3W3

Patrick Lachance
Regional Administrator
South Shore Regional Office
P.O. Box 1360
Liverpool, Nova Scotia
B0T 1K0

Elaine MacPherson
Clerk-Treasurer
P.O. Box 88
Louisbourg, Nova Scotia
B0A 1M0

Cyril Reddy
Regional Administrator
North Shore Regional Office
P.O. Box 488
New Glasgow, Nova Scotia
B2H 5E5

Bernard MacNeil
Director of Social Services
3371 Plummer Avenue
New Waterford, Nova Scotia
B1H 1Y8

Keith MacMillan
Social Service Worker
262 Commercial Street
Box 369
North Sydney, Nova Scotia
B2A 3M4

Harris M. McCormack
Clerk-Treasurer
P.O. Box 338
Oxford, Nova Scotia
B0M 1P0

Gordon MacMaster
District Supervisor
P.O. Box 359
Port Hawkesbury, Nova Scotia
B0E 2V0

Beverly MacLeod
Director of Social Services
P.O. Box 2549
Springhill, Nova Scotia
B0M 1X0

Pat Drohan
Director of Social Services
P.O. Box 730
Sydney, Nova Scotia
B1P 6H7

Harvey MacArthur
Executive Director
P.O. Box 950
Truro, Nova Scotia
B2N 5G7

Wendy Trull
District Supervisor
P.O. Box 2350
Windsor, Nova Scotia
B0N 2T0

Mike Kendrick
Acting Regional Administrator
Western Regional Office
P.O. Box 460
Yarmouth, Nova Scotia
B5A 4B5

OCCUPATIONAL THERAPISTS

Nova Scotia Association of
Occupational Therapists (NSAOT)
P.O. Box 3082
Halifax South
Halifax, Nova Scotia
B3J 3G6

Nova Scotia Society of Occupational
Therapists (NSSOT)
P.O. Box 3082
Halifax South
Halifax, Nova Scotia
B3J 3G6
464-3116

THE PARKINSON FOUNDATION OF CANADA

Halifax, Nova Scotia
454-2468
424-1887

Sydney, Nova Scotia
564-4335

Truro, Nova Scotia
895-7238
893-2213
519-979-3082

RED CROSS

Canadian Red Cross Society
Nova Scotia
1940 Gottingen Street
P.O. Box 366
Halifax, Nova Scotia
B3J 2H2

SELF-HELP CLEARING HOUSES

The Self Help Connection
5739 Inglis Street
Halifax, Nova Scotia
B3H 1K5
422-5831

SELF-HELP GROUPS

Alzheimer Society of Nova Scotia
5954 Spring Garden Road
Halifax, Nova Scotia
B3H 1Y7
422-7961

Alzheimer Society of Nova Scotia
"Seniors"
P.O. Box 3413
Bayers Road Shopping Centre
Halifax, Nova Scotia
443-0695

Canadian Pensioners Concerned Inc.—
Womens Committee
Tower 1, Suite 103
Halifax Shopping Centre
7001 Mumford Road
Halifax, Nova Scotia
B3L 2H9
455-7684

Community Contact for the Widowed
6366 Pepperell Street
Halifax, Nova Scotia
B3H 2P4
422-5609

Dartmouth Share
45 Octerloney Street
Box 1146
Dartmouth, Nova Scotia
B2Y 4B8
465-5578

Dartmouth Stroke Club
Findlay Recreation Centre
26 Elliot Street
P.O. Box 817
Dartmouth, Nova Scotia
463-5269/421-2228

Friendship in Action
45 Octerloney Street
Dartmouth, Nova Scotia
B2Y 4M7
465-5578

Metro Volunteer Resource Centre
Halifax Metro Volunteer Resource
Centre
P.O. Box 5066
Armdale, Nova Scotia
B3L 4M6
423-1368

Multiple Sclerosis Society of Canada—
Atlantic Division
Suite 612
45 Alderney Drive
Dartmouth, Nova Scotia
B2Y 2N6
465-7251

Nova Scotia Heart Foundation
321-1657 Barrington Street
P.O. Box 1585
Halifax, Nova Scotia
B3J 2Y3
423-7530

Parkinson's Disease—Seniors
Committee
5954 Spring Garden Road
Halifax, Nova Scotia
422-7919

Senior Citizens Matinee Group
3621 Robie Street
Halifax, Nova Scotia
B3K 4S8
455-0921

Senior Citizens Secretariat
424-0065 (toll free)

Senior Committee of Metro Halifax
Ostomy Association
Visitation and Workshops
3 Berkeley Brae
Dartmouth, Nova Scotia
B2Y 4G6

Senior Committee of Metro Halifax
Ostomy Association
6215 Cedar Street
Halifax, Nova Scotia
B3H 2K1

Seniors Newsletter
#203-166 Cowie Hill Road
Halifax, Nova Scotia
B3P 2N8
479-3514 (after 6:00 p.m.)

Spencer House Seniors Centre
5596 Morris Street
Halifax, Nova Scotia
B3J 1C2
421-6131

The Volunteer Centre of Halifax
511 Young Avenue
Halifax, Nova Scotia
B3H 2V4

NEW BRUNSWICK

CANADIAN MENTAL HEALTH ASSOCIATION

Ms. Donna Cormier
CMHA—Region VIII
C P 412
Campbellton, New Brunswick
E3N 3G7

CMHA—N.B. Division
Region V
P.O. Box 412
Campbellton, New Brunswick
E3N 1B1
759-9777

CMHA—N.B. Division
Region VII
337 Water Street
Chatham, New Brunswick
E1N 1B2
773-7561

Ms. Anne Marie Hartford
CMHA—Region XI
362 Water Street
Chatham, New Brunswick
E1N 1B5
773-7561

CMHA—N.B. Division
Region IV
11 Costisan
P.O. Box 333
Edmunston, New Brunswick
E3V 1W7
739-9489

Ms. Denyse Martin
CMHA—Region VII
28e, rue St-Francois
Edmunston, New Brunswick
E3V 1R9

CMHA—N.B. Division
Suite 214, 65 Brunswick Street
Fredericton, New Brunswick
E3B 1G5
455-5231

Jean McBrine, Coordinator
CMHA—Central N.B. Branch
65 Brunswick Street, Room 254
Fredericton, New Brunswick
E3B 1G5
458-1803

CMHA—N.B. Division
Region III
Room 260, 65 Brunswick Street
Fredericton, New Brunswick
E3B 1G5
458-9155

Ms. Sherry Lapointe
CMHA—Region V, VI
Victoria Health Centre
65 Brunswick Street
Fredericton, New Brunswick
E3B 1G5

Mrs. Susan Davenport
Executive Director
CMHA—Moncton Branch
P.O. Box 11
Moncton, New Brunswick
E1C 8R9
859-8114

Regional Community Worker
CMHA—Region I, II
495 Elmwood Drive, Apt. 21
Moncton, New Brunswick
E1A 2B4

CMHA—N.B. Division
Region I
P.O. Box 719
Richibouctou, New Brunswick
E0A 2M0
523-7112

CMHA—N.B. Division
Saint John Branch
Suite 1036
400 Main Street
Saint John, New Brunswick
E2K 1J4
633-1705

CMHA—N.B. Division
Region II
Suite 1036
400 Main Street
Saint John, New Brunswick
E2K 1J4
634-7225

Ms. Kathy Crowell
CMHA—Region III, IV
Place 400
400 Main Street
Saint John, New Brunswick
E2K 1J4

CMHA—N.B. Division
Region VI
P.O. Box 753
Shippagan, New Brunswick
E0B 2P0
336-4932

Ms. Lucie Robichaud
CMHA—Region IX, X
C P 753
178, rue Hotel de Ville
Shippagan, New Brunswick
C0B 2P0

CANADIAN NATIONAL INSTITUTE FOR THE BLIND

Northern Regional Office
700 St. Peter Avenue
Bathurst, New Brunswick
E2A 2Y7
546-9922

P.O. Box 550
55 Emmerson Street
Edmundston, New Brunswick
E3V 3L2
739-9533

390 King Street
Fredericton, New Brunswick
E3B 1E3
458-0060

118 Highfield Street
Moncton, New Brunswick
E1C 5N7
857-4240

350 Morrison Lane
P.O. Box 296
Newcastle, New Brunswick
E1V 2C1
622-1513

Southern Regional Office
33 Beaverbrook Avenue
Saint John, New Brunswick
E2K 2W2
634-7277

CANADIAN PARAPLEGIC ASSOCIATION—N.B. DIVISION

Educational and Employment Services
2nd Floor
216 Main Street
Bathurst, New Brunswick
E2A 1A8
548-5700

32-17th Street
Edmundston, New Brunswick
E3V 2L5
739-8988

Rehab Programs/Services
65 Brunswick Street
Fredericton, New Brunswick
E3B 1G5
458-1189

Educational and Employment Services
Suite 209
95 Foundry Street
Moncton, New Brunswick
E1C 5H7
858-0311

Regional Rehabilitation Services
Department of Health & Community
Services
P.O. Box 7000
Newcastle, New Brunswick
E1V 3N3

Educational and Employment Services
P.O. Box 2549
Saint John, New Brunswick
E2L 4S8
648-9103

COMMUNITY-BASED SERVICES FOR DISABLED PERSONS

Department of Health and
Community Services
P.O. Box 5001
165 St. Andrew Street
Bathurst, New Brunswick
E2A 3Z9
547-2020

Department of Health and
Community Services
4th Floor
City Centre Mall
Water Street
P.O. Box 5001
Campbellton, New Brunswick
E3N 3H5
759-8861

Department of Health and
Community Services
433 Edifice Rona
Place St. Pierre
St. Pierre Boulevard
P.O. Box 5001
Caraquet, New Brunswick
E0B 1K0
727-4455

Department of Health and
Community Services
276 Water Street
P.O. Box 5001
Chatham, New Brunswick
E1N 1B1
773-5841

Department of Health and
Community Services
Woodlawn Avenue
P.O. Box 5001
Dorchester, New Brunswick
E0A 1M0
379-2411

Department of Health and
Community Services
Carrefour Assomption
Church Street
P.O. Box 5001
Edmundston, New Brunswick
E3V 3L3
739-6651

Department of Health and
Community Services
300 St. Mary's Street
P.O. Box 5001
Fredericton, New Brunswick
E3B 5G8
453-3953

Department of Health and
Community Services
166 Broadway
P.O. Box 5001
Grand Falls, New Brunswick
E0J 1M0
473-6210

Department of Health and
Community Services
2nd Floor
Provincial Building
Notre Dame Street
P.O. Box 27
Kedgwick, New Brunswick
E0K 1C0
284-3038

Department of Health and
Community Services
Assomption Place
770 Main Street
P.O. Box 5001
Moncton, New Brunswick
E1C 8R3
856-2400

Department of Health and
Community Services
Main Street
P.O. Box 5001
Neguac, New Brunswick
E0C 1S0
776-8347

Department of Health and
Community Services
McCombs Building
Henry Street
P.O. Box 7000
Newcastle, New Brunswick
E1V 3N3
622-8762

Department of Health and
Community Services
Main Street
P.O. Box 5001
Perth-Andover, New Brunswick
E0J 1V0
273-2059

Department of Health and
Community Services
Cartier Mall
Alder Street
P.O. Box 5001
Richibucto, New Brunswick
E0A 2M0
523-4431

Department of Health and
Community Services
8 Castle Street
P.O. Box 2900
Saint John, New Brunswick
E2L 5A3
658-2734

Department of Health and
Community Services
2nd Floor
Centreville Mall
Main Street
P.O. Box 1210
Shediac, New Brunswick
E0A 3G0
532-6608

Department of Health and
Community Services
Dominique Gauthier Building
P.O. Box 5001
Shippagan, New Brunswick
E0B 2P0
336-8469

Department of Health and
Community Services
2nd Floor
Provincial Building
41 King Street
P.O. Box 5001
St. Stephen, New Brunswick
E3L 2X4
466-4260

Department of Health and
Community Services
1st Floor
Provincial Building
Main Street
P.O. Box 5001
Sussex, New Brunswick
E0E 1P0
432-2004

Department of Health and
Community Services
Place Tracadie, rue Principale
Tracadie, New Brunswick
E0C 2B0
395-6391

Department of Health and
Community Services
Bicentennial Building
200 King Street
P.O. Box 5001
Woodstock, New Brunswick
E0J 2B0
328-9251

FAMILY SERVICE CANADA

Family Enrichment & Counselling
Services
618 Queen Street
Fredericton, New Brunswick
E3B 1C2
458-8211

Family Service Moncton, Inc.
386 St. George Street
Moncton, New Brunswick
E1C 1X2
857-3258

Family Services Saint John Inc.
369 Rockland Road
Saint John, New Brunswick
E2K 3W3
634-8295

Service de Counselling et
d'Enrichissement Familial, Inc.
235 Main Street
Bathurst, New Brunswick
E2A 1A9
546-3305

Service de counselling et
d'enrichissement familial, Inc.
29 rue Aqueduc
Edmundston, Nouveau Brunswick
E3V 1X7
735-3325

MEALS ON WHEELS

101 St. Patrick Street
Atholville, New Brunswick

500 Queen Street
Bathurst, New Brunswick

P.O. Box 149
Boisetown, New Brunswick

180 Upper Water Street
Chatham, New Brunswick

Chipman, New Brunswick

Canadian Red Cross
128 Church Street
Edmundston, New Brunswick

65 Brunswick Street
Fredericton, New Brunswick

White Rapids Manor
Fredericton Junction, New Brunswick

P.O. Box 130
Gagetown, New Brunswick

Canadian Red Cross
P.O. Box 112
Grand Falls, New Brunswick

Harvey Community Hospital
Harvey Station, New Brunswick

MacLean Memorial Hospital
Saunders Road
McAdam, New Brunswick

42 Silver Lane
Moncton, New Brunswick

3 Cavendish Road
Moncton, New Brunswick

Health & Community Services
65 Henry Street
Newcastle, New Brunswick

519 Gardiner Street
Oromocto, New Brunswick

Tobique Valley Manor
Plaster Rock, New Brunswick

Minto Meals on Wheels
R.R. #1
Ripples, New Brunswick

P.O. Box 7091
Station "A"
Saint John, New Brunswick

P.O. Box 5001
Shippagan, New Brunswick

St. Andrews Health Clinic
St. Andrews, New Brunswick

Health & Community Services
P.O. Box 5001
St. Stephen, New Brunswick

P.O. Box 194
Stanley, New Brunswick

Canadian Red Cross
38 Maple Street
Sussex, New Brunswick

P.O. Box 458
Tracadie, New Brunswick

P.O. Box 1388
Woodstock, New Brunswick

OCCUPATIONAL THERAPISTS

New Brunswick Association of
Occupational Therapists (NBAOT)
c/o Forest Hill Rehabilitation Centre
180 Woodbridge Street
Fredericton, New Brunswick
E3B 4R3
458-8353

New Brunswick Association of
Occupational Therapists (NBAOT)
c/o Workers Rehabilitation Centre
P.O. Box 3067, Postal Stn. B
St. John, New Brunswick
E2M 4X7
738-8411

THE PARKINSON FOUNDATION OF CANADA

Fredericton, New Brunswick
458-8353

Moncton, New Brunswick
384-3567

Riverview, New Brunswick
386-7356

Saint John, New Brunswick
693-9842
633-3100
633-2675
657-3231
833-2235

RED CROSS

Canadian Red Cross Society
New Brunswick
405 University Avenue
P.O. Box 39
Saint John, New Brunswick
E2L 3X3
648-5000; 1-800-561-9151

SELF-HELP GROUPS

Adult Day Centre
c/o VON
65 Brunswick Street
Fredericton, New Brunswick
E3B 1G5
458-8365

Alzheimer Society of Canada
Provincial Office
P.O. Box 3126, Station "B"
Fredericton, New Brunswick
E3A 5G9
453-0892

Alzheimer Society of New Brunswick
Suite 201
Victoria Health Centre
65 Brunswick Street
Fredericton, New Brunswick
E3B 1G5
453-0892

Amyotrophic Lateral Sclerosis Society
of New Brunswick Inc.
P.O. Box 295
Moncton, New Brunswick
E1C 8K9
855-1239

The Arthritis Society—N.B. Division
Victoria Health Centre
65 Brunswick Street
Fredericton, New Brunswick
E3B 1G5
454-6114

L'Association Des Handicapes Physiques
De La Peninsule Acadienne, Inc.
643 Boulevard St-Pierre West
Caraquet, New Brunswick
E0B 1K0
727-6095 or 764-5592

L'Association Des Handicapes
Physiques De La Region De Tracadie
P.O. Box 335
Tracadie, New Brunswick
E0C 2B0
395-9242, 395-5728 or 395-3924

Bathurst Volunteer Centre de bénévolat
Local 3E
159 Main Street
Bathurst, New Brunswick
E2A 3Z9
546-9879

Canadian Council for the Blind—
Maritime Division
175 St. Patrick Street
Bathurst, New Brunswick
E2A 1C8
548-2621

Canadian Cystic Fibrosis Foundation
33 d'Amour Street
Edmundston, New Brunswick
E3V 1Y1
735-4465

Canadian Cystic Fibrosis Foundation
P.O. Box 115
Grand Bay, New Brunswick
E0G 1W0
738-8996

Canadian Cystic Fibrosis Foundation
105-1/2 High Street
Moncton, New Brunswick
E1C 6B6
854-5549

Canadian Cystic Fibrosis Foundation
220 Alexander Street
Newcastle, New Brunswick
E1V 1H3
622-8858

Canadian Cystic Fibrosis Foundation
General Delivery
Woodstock, New Brunswick
E0J 2B0
328-6065

Canadian Rehabilitation Council for
the Disabled—N.B. Branch Inc.
65 Brunswick Street
Fredericton, New Brunswick
E3B 1G5
458-8739

Le Centre régional de bénévolat de la
Peninsule acadienne
P.O. Box 397
Caraquet, New Brunswick
E0B 1K0
727-2582

Cerebral Palsy Association
24 Bristol Street
Fredericton, New Brunswick
E3B 4W3
454-2804

Cerebral Palsy Foundation, Inc.
P.O. Box 2152
Saint John, New Brunswick
E2L 3V1
635-8932

CHIMO Help Centre, Inc.
P.O. Box 1033
Fredericton, New Brunswick
E3B 5C2
450-4357; TDD 450-7046

COIL Inc.
Centres Offering Independent
Lifestyles
P.O. Box 2273
Saint John, New Brunswick
E2L 3V1
847-5895

Department of Health and
Community Services
P.O. Box 5100
Fredericton, New Brunswick
E3B 5G8
453-2843; TDD 453-7167

Department of Transportation
Transportation & Communications
Policy
Room 282
York Tower
Kings Place
P.O. Box 6000
Fredericton, New Brunswick
E3B 5H1
453-2802

Dial-A-Bus
City of Fredericton
Transit Department
P.O. Box 130
Fredericton, New Brunswick
E3B 4Y7
458-9522

Extra-Mural Hospital
Acadian Peninsula Unit
3507 Main Street
P.O. Box 6000
Racadie, New Brunswick
E0C 2B0
395-6357

Extra-Mural Hospital
Bathurst Unit
P.O. Box 1226
Bathurst, New Brunswick
E2A 4J1
548-4555

Extra-Mural Hospital
Blance Bourgeois Unit
Francophone Unit
835 Champlain Street
Dieppe, New Brunswick
E1A 1P6
857-8066

Extra-Mural Hospital
Driscoll Unit
English Unit
84 Driscoll Crescent
Moncton, New Brunswick
E1E 3R8
857-8047

Extra-Mural Hospital
Edmundston Unit
174 Hebert Boulevard
Edmundston, New Brunswick
E3V 2S7
735-0160

Extra-Mural Hospital
Fredericton Unit
200 Prospect Street West
Fredericton, New Brunswick
E3B 2T8
458-0120

Extra-Mural Hospital
Grand Falls Unit
P.O. Box 2559
Grand Falls, New Brunswick
E0J 1M0
473-5192

Extra-Mural Hospital
Miramichi Unit
296 Radio Street
Newcastle, New Brunswick
E1V 2W5
622-2498

Extra-Mural Hospital
Saint John & Kennebecasis Unit
Marr Road
P.O. Box 670
Rothesay, New Brunswick
E0G 2W0
847-9826

Extra-Mural Hospital
Shediac Unit
P.O. Box 150
Pointe-du-Chêne, New Brunswick
E0A 2J0
532-9700

Extra-Mural Hospital
St. Stephen Unit
P.O. Box 483
St. Stephen, New Brunswick
E3L 1G0
466-6073

Extra-Mural Hospital
Sussex Unit
P.O. Box 870
Sussex, Ontario
E0E 1P0
433-1744

Extra-Mural Hospital
Woodstock Unit
Nurses' Residence
P.O. Box 2019
Woodstock, New Brunswick
E0J 2B0
328-9318

Family Enrichment & Counselling
Services (Fredericton) Inc.
618 Queen Street
Fredericton, New Brunswick
E3B 1C2
458-8211

Family Enrichment & Counselling
Services, Inc.
29 Aqueduc Street
Edmundston, New Brunswick
E3V 1X7
735-3325

Family and Friends
78 Weldon Street
Moncton, New Brunswick
E1C 8R9
859-8114

Family Service Moncton Inc.
386 St. George Street
Moncton, New Brunswick
E1C 1X2

Family Services Nepisiguit Inc.
235 Main Street
Bathurst, New Brunswick
E2A 1A9
546-3305

Family Services (Sussex) Inc.
689 Main Street
P.O. Box 669
Sussex, New Brunswick
E0E 1P0
433-5959

Fredericton Association for the Deaf
592 Doone Street
Fredericton, New Brunswick
E3A 2S6
472-9211

Fredericton Stroke Club
UNB Faculty of Nursing
Fredericton, New Brunswick
E3B 5A3
453-4642

Info-Line
Saint John Human Development
Council
P.O. Box 6125, Station "A"
Saint John, New Brunswick
E2L 4R6
633-4636

Kidney Foundation of Canada
Victoria Health Centre
65 Brunswick Street
Fredericton, New Brunswick
E3B 1G5
454-6690

Ministry to the Deaf
Wesleyan Church
P.O. Box 1206
Moncton, New Brunswick
E1C 8P9
854-1320 or 384-7384

Miramichi Physically Disabled &
Handicapped Association, Inc.
2 Johnson Street
Chatham, New Brunswick
E1N 3B7
773-9437

The Miramichi Volunteer Services
Bureau, Inc.
P.O. Box 249
Chatham, New Brunswick
E1N 3A7
773-9549 or 622-2800

Moncton Association for the Deaf
31 Garland Drive
Riverview, New Brunswick
E1B 3V3
TTY 386-8091

Moncton Community Residences, Inc.
357 Collishaw Street
P.O. Box 2875, Station "A"
Moncton, New Brunswick
E1C 8T8
858-0550

Moncton Respite Care Services
Suite 406
236 St. George Street
Moncton, New Brunswick
E1C 1W1
857-8361

Moncton Volunteer Centre du
bénévolat
236 St. George Street
Moncton, New Brunswick
E1C 1V9
857-8005 or 857-8009

Multiple Sclerosis Society of Canada—
Atlantic Division
Restigouche County
11 Esquadich Road
Campbellton, New Brunswick
E3N 2E5

Multiple Sclerosis Society of Canada—
Atlantic Division
Fredericton
Apartment 416
570 Aberdeen Street
Fredericton, New Brunswick
E3B 5N4

Multiple Sclerosis Society of Canada—
Atlantic Division
Moncton
211 Bond Drive
Moncton, New Brunswick
E1E 1A1

Multiple Sclerosis Society of Canada—
Atlantic Division
Saint John
P.O. Box 654
Saint John, New Brunswick
E2L 2W0

Multiple Sclerosis Society of Canada—
Atlantic Division
Kings County
P.O. Box 1265
Sussex, New Brunswick
E0E 1P0

The Muscular Dystrophy Association
of Canada
Provincial Office
281 Restigouche Road
Ormocto, New Brunswick
E2V 2H2
446-6322

Neil Squire Foundation
65 Brunswick Street
Fredericton, New Brunswick
E3B 1G5
450-7999

New Brunswick Association for
Community Living
86 York Street
Fredericton, New Brunswick
E3B 3N5
458-8866

New Brunswick Association of
Occupational Therapists
The Registrar
O.T. Department
Forest Hill Rehabilitation Centre
180 Woodbridge Street
Fredericton, New Brunswick
E3B 4R3
458-8353

New Brunswick Association of
Physiotherapists
P.O. Box 1234
Fredericton, New Brunswick
328-3391

New Brunswick Coordinating Council
on Deafness
206 Winslow Street
Saint John, New Brunswick
E2M 1W8
672-2778

New Brunswick Extra-Mural Hospital
200 Prospect Street West
Fredericton, New Brunswick
E3B 2T8
458-8630

New Brunswick Heart and Stroke
Foundation
61 King Street
Saint John, New Brunswick
E2L 1G5
634-1620

New Brunswick Senior Citizens'
Federation Inc.
Place Heritage Court
421-95 Foundry Street
Moncton, New Brunswick
E1C 5H7
857-8242

Office of the Ombudsman
703 Brunswick Street
P.O. Box 6000
Fredericton, New Brunswick
E3B 5H1
453-2789; 1-800-561-4021

Opal III Respite Services
1188 Woodstock Road
Comp. 8, Site 1, R.R. #3
Fredericton, New Brunswick
E3B 4X4

Oromocto Information Service Centre/
Volunteer Bureau
68 Iroquois Avenue
Oromocto, New Brunswick
E2V 2G6
357-9494 Volunteer Bureau; 357-8888
Info Line

Parkinson Foundation of Canada
Health & Community Services
P.O. Box 5001
Fredericton, New Brunswick
E3B 5G4
453-2825

Parkinson Foundation of Canada
Seniors' Outreach Centre
Loch Lomond Villa
185 Loch Lomond Road
Saint John, New Brunswick
E2J 3S3
633-2675, ext. 640

People Care Inc.
65 Brunswick Street
Fredericton, New Brunswick
E3B 1G5
453-9192

Saint John Association of the Deaf
55 Canterbury Street
Saint John, New Brunswick
E2L 2C6
634-7340 TDD only

Saint John Hearing Society
Hilyard Place
3rd Floor, Building "A"
560 Main Street
Saint John, New Brunswick
E2K 1J5
633-0599 or 633-0796 (voice and TDD)

Saint John Stroke Club
P.O. Box 3214, Station "B"
Saint John, New Brunswick
E2M 4X8
672-7918

Saint John Volunteer Centre, Inc.
P.O. Box 7091, Station "A"
Saint John, New Brunswick
E2L 4S5

Seniors' Outreach Centre
Loch Lomond Villa Inc.
185 Loch Lomond Road
Saint John, New Brunswick
E2J 3S3
633-2675, ext. 640

Services Communautaires De L'Arc Inc.
P.O. Box 134
Rogersville, New Brunswick
E0A 2T0
775-2583 or 775-6529

St. John Ambulance
P.O. Box 3599, Station "B"
Fredericton, New Brunswick
E3A 5J8
458-9129

St. Stephen Volunteer Centre, Inc.
199 Union Street
St. Stephen, New Brunswick
E3L 2W9
466-4995

Tel-Aide Information Centre
Tel-Aide Listens Inc.
55 Emmerson Street
Edmundston, New Brunswick
E3V 1R9
739-7218; 1-800-222-9543

Tel-Aide Listens Inc.
P. O. Box 687
Edmunston, New Brunswick
E3V 1R9
739-6307; 1-800-222-9543

United Way Volunteer Bureau of
Fredericton, Inc.
65 Brunswick Street
Fredericton, New Brunswick
E3B 1G5
452-8595

Victorian Order of Nurses
Bathurst Branch
P.O. Box 213
Bathurst, New Brunswick
E2A 3Z2
548-2448

Victorian Order of Nurses
Campbellton Branch
P.O. Box 742
Campbellton, New Brunswick
E3N 3H2
753-4750

Victorian Order of Nurses
Edmundston Branch
Suite 208
55 Emmerson Street
Edmundston, New Brunswick
E3V 1R9
739-6318

Victorian Order of Nurses
Fredericton Branch
65 Brunswick Street
Fredericton, New Brunswick
E3B 1G5
458-8365

Victorian Order of Nurses
Miramichi Branch
41A Lobban Avenue
Chatham, New Brunswick
E1N 2W8
773-9622

Victorian Order of Nurses
Moncton Branch
Suite 300
96 Norwood Avenue
Moncton, New Brunswick
E1C 6L9
857-9115

Victorian Order of Nurses
Oromocto Branch
137 MacDonald Avenue
Oromocto, New Brunswick
E2V 1A6
357-8542

Victorian Order of Nurses
Sackville Branch
P.O. Box 75
Sackville, New Brunswick
E0A 3C0
536-0750

Victorian Order of Nurses
Saint John Branch
439 Prince Street West
Saint John, New Brunswick
E2M 1R2
635-1530

Victorian Order of Nurses
Woodstock Branch
P.O. Box 1096
Woodstock, New Brunswick
E0J 2B0
328-8224

Volunteer Bureau
P.O. Box 7091, Station "A"
Saint John, New Brunswick
E2L 4S5

PRINCE EDWARD ISLAND

CANADIAN MENTAL HEALTH ASSOCIATION

Mr. Allan James
Executive Director
CMHA—Prince Edward Island Division
170 Fitzroy Street
P.O. Box 785
Charlottetown, Prince Edward Island
C1A 7L9

FAMILY SERVICE CANADA

Catholic Family Services Bureau
P.O. Box 698
129 Pownal Street
Charlottetown, Prince Edward Island
C1A 7L3
894-8591

Protestant Family Service Bureau
216 Queen Street
P.O. Box 592
Charlottetown, Prince Edward Island
C1A 8C1
892-2441

OCCUPATIONAL THERAPISTS

Prince Edward Island Association of
Occupational Therapists (PEIAOT)
P.O. Box 2248
Charlottetown, Prince Edward Island
C1A 8B9
368-5023

Prince Edward Island Occupational
Therapy Society (PEIOTS)
P.O. Box 2248
Charlottetown, Prince Edward Island
C1A 8B9
838-2772

RED CROSS

Canadian Red Cross Society
Prince Edward Island
62 Prince Street
Charlottetown, Prince Edward Island
C1A 4R2

SELF-HELP GROUPS

Alzheimer Society of P.E.I.
R.R. #2
N. Wiltshire, Prince Edward Island
C0A 1Y0
964-2780

Community Care Facilities and
Nursing Homes Board
P.O. Box 2000
Charlottetown, Prince Edward Island
C1A 7N8

Heart and Stroke Foundation of Prince
Edward Island
40 Queen Street
Charlottetown, Prince Edward Island
C1A 7K4
892-7441

Nursing Home Association of P.E.I.
16 Centennial Drive
Charlottetown, Prince Edward Island
C1A 6C5
566-5975

P.E.I. Association on Gerontology
P.O. Box 3346
Charlottetown, Prince Edward Island
C1A 8W5

P.E.I. Seniors Federation
25 Lapthorne Avenue
Charlottetown, Prince Edward Island
C1A 2M3
368-7070

Senior Resource Group
5 Royal Court
Charlottetown, Prince Edward Island
C1A 8M7
894-4228

Seniors' Infoline
368-7538

Volunteer Resource Council
81 Prince Street
Charlottetown, Prince Edward Island
C1A 4R3
892-3790

VISITING HOMEMAKER SERVICE, HOME CARE AND SUPPORT

Charlottetown, Prince Edward Island
894-7332

Montague, Prince Edward Island
838-2992

O'Leary, Prince Edward Island
859-2400

Souris, Prince Edward Island
687-3022

Summerside, Prince Edward Island
463-2169/436-2160

NEWFOUNDLAND

ADULT DAY CARE PROGRAMS

Brookfield Hospital
Valleyfield, B.B., Newfoundland
536-2406

Carmelite House
Grand Falls, Newfoundland
489-2274

ASSESSMENT SERVICES

L.A. Miller Centre
St. John's, Newfoundland
737-7367

CANADIAN MENTAL HEALTH ASSOCIATION

Mr. Phillip Walters
Branch Staff Contact
CMHA—Corner Brook Region Branch
171 Eastvalley Road
Cornerbrook, Newfoundland
A2H 2M1

Ms. Beverly Dawson
Branch Staff Contact
CMHA—Gander Region Branch
18 Alrock Crescent
Gander, Newfoundland
A1V 1K4

DAY HOSPITALS

Division of Services to Senior Citizens
Department of Health
P.O. Box 8700
St. John's, Newfoundland
A1B 4J6

L.A. Miller Centre
c/o Department of Health's
Co-ordinator of Placements
St. John's, Newfoundland

Lakeside Homes
Gander, Newfoundland
256-8850

Lion's Manor
Placentia, Newfoundland
227-2061

North Haven Manor
Lewisporte, Newfoundland
535-6726

Paddon Memorial Home
Happy Valley, Newfoundland

Saint Luke's Homes
St. John's, Newfoundland
579-0052

St. Anthony Interfaith Home
St. Anthony, Newfoundland
454-3506

Valley Vista
Springdale, Newfoundland
673-3936

FAMILY SERVICE CANADA

The Family Life Bureau, St. John's
P.O. Box 4364
St. John's, Newfoundland
A1C 5S5
579-0168

HOME CARE PROGRAMS

Geriatric Medical Clinic
L.A. Miller Centre
St. John's, Newfoundland
737-7370

Geriatric Psychiatric Clinic
L.A. Miller Centre
St. John's, Newfoundland
737-6717

HOME HELP—HOMEMAKING SERVICES

Social Services District Office
Department of Social Services

Gander & District Continuing
Care Program
Gander, Newfoundland
256-7969

Golden Heights Manor
Bonavista, Newfoundland
468-2043

Harry L. Paddon Memorial Home
Happy Valley, Newfoundland
896-2469

Labrador South Home Care
Forteau, Newfoundland
931-2450

LeGrow Hospital
Channel, Newfoundland
695-2151

St. John's Home Care Program (Metro)
St. John's, Newfoundland
753-3095

Valley Vista Senior Citizens Home
Springdale, Newfoundland
673-3936

MEAL SERVICES

Bay St. George Senior Citizens Home
Stephenville Crossing, Newfoundland
646-2732

Blue Crest Interfaith Home
Grand Bank, Newfoundland
832-1660

Community Services Council
P.O. Box #5116
Virginia Park Plaza
Newfoundland Drive
St. John's, Newfoundland
A1C 5Z3
753-9860

Conception-Trinity Interfaith Home
Carbonear, Newfoundland
596-5101

Harbour Lodge
c/o Department of Health's
Co-ordinator of Placements
St. John's, Newfoundland

Hoyles/Escansoni Complex
c/o Department of Health's
Co-ordinator of Placements
St. John's, Newfoundland

Hugh Twomey Health Care Centre
Botwood, Newfoundland

J.J. O'Connell Centre
Corner Brook, Newfoundland
637-5000

Victorian Order of Nurses
St. John's, Newfoundland
726-8597

OCCUPATIONAL THERAPY

Newfoundland and Labrador
Association of Occupational Therapists
(NLAOT)
P.O. Box 5423
St. John's, Newfoundland
A1C 5W2
364-0325

Newfoundland and Labrador
Occupational Therapy Board (NLOTB)
P.O. Box 7203
Westend Post Office
St. John's, Newfoundland
A1E 3Y4

THE PARKINSON FOUNDATION OF CANADA

St. John's, Newfoundland
722-0621

RED CROSS

Canadian Red Cross Society
Newfoundland & Labrador
7 Wicklow Street
P.O. Box 13156, Station "A"
St. John's, Newfoundland
A1B 4A4

RESPITE CARE SERVICES

Heart and Stroke Foundation of
Newfoundland and Labrador
P.O. Box 5819
St. John's, Newfoundland
A1C 5X3

Newfoundland Alzheimer
Association Inc.
Suite 328-329, 3rd Floor
Southcott Hall
100 Forest Road
St. John's, Newfoundland
A1A 1E5
576-0608

SELF-HELP GROUPS

Bay St. George Senior Citizens Home
Stephenville Crossing, Newfoundland
646-2732

Bonnews Lodge
Valleyfield, Newfoundland
536-2160

Conception-Trinity Interfaith Home
Carbonear, Newfoundland
596-5101

Golden Heights Manor
Bonavista, Newfoundland
468-2043

Lakeside Homes
Gander, Newfoundland
256-8850

LeGrow Hospital
Channel, Newfoundland
695-2151

North Haven Manor
Lewisporte, Newfoundland
535-6726

Saint Luke's Homes
St. John's, Newfoundland
579-0052

St. Anthony Interfaith Home
St. Anthony, Newfoundland
454-3506

V.O.N. Adult Day Care
29 Wellington Street
Corner Brook, Newfoundland

YUKON

CANADIAN MENTAL HEALTH ASSOCIATION

Mr. Charles Pugh
Executive Director
CMHA—Yukon Division
8 Green Crescent
Whitehorse, Yukon
Y1A 4RN

RED CROSS

Canadian Red Cross Society
British Columbia–Yukon
4710 Kingsway
Suite 400
Burnaby, British Columbia
V5H 4M2

SELF-HELP GROUPS

Seniors Information Centre
#3-106 Main Street
Whitehorse, Yukon
Y1A 2A8
668-3383

Yukon Association for
Community Living
106 Main Street
Whitehorse, Yukon
Y1A 2A8
667-4606

Yukon Territorial Government
Department of Health and
Human Resources
Seniors Services
Yukon Homecare Program
Box 2703
Whitehorse, Yukon
Y1A 2C6
667-5674; 1-800-661-0408

NORTHWEST TERRITORIES

CANADIAN MENTAL HEALTH ASSOCIATION

Inuvik Branch
Box 1915
Inuvik, North West Territories
X0E 0T0